Ladies Weight Loss Programme

Parvesh Handa

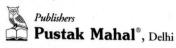

Publishers
Pustak Mahal®, Delhi

J-3/16 , Daryaganj, New Delhi-110002
☎ 23276539, 23272783, 23272784 • *Fax:* 011-23260518
E-mail: info@pustakmahal.com • *Website:* www.pustakmahal.com

London Office
51, Severn Crescents, Slough, Berkshire, SL 38 UU, England
E-mail: pustakmahaluk@pustakmahal.com

Sales Centre
10-B, Netaji Subhash Marg, Daryaganj, New Delhi-110002
☎ 23268292, 23268293, 23279900 • *Fax:* 011-23280567
E-mail: rapidexdelhi@indiatimes.com

Branch Offices
Bangalore: ☎ 22234025
E-mail: pmblr@sancharnet.in • pustak@sancharnet.in
Mumbai: ☎ 22010941
E-mail: rapidex@bom5.vsnl.net.in
Patna: ☎ 3294193 • *Telefax:* 0612-2302719
E-mail: rapidexptn@rediffmail.com
Hyderabad: *Telefax:* 040-24737290
E-mail: pustakmahalhyd@yahoo.co.in

© Author

ISBN 978-81-223-0985-0

Edition : January 2008

Printed at : Param Offsetters, Okhla, New Delhi-110020

NOTICE
This book is a reference only, not a medical guide or manual of self-treatment.
No treatment should be taken without consultation of a doctor.

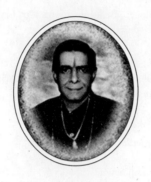

Lovingly dedicated to

Respected Guru Dev

Dr. Pt. Manmohan Shastri Ji

of Babyal, Ambala Cantt.

for his constant Gifts of Light, Life, Inspirations

&

Divine True Love

A few words about this book

If you want to slim down and stay attractive and healthy – then this is the book for you.

It is a programme that will guide you gently into a new way of eating that does not unbalance your body. This book describes how you may control ageing and keep your body fit with the help of various techniques: simple movements, yoga, massage, exercise and gymnastics, and latest medical facts on diet and nutrition, without unpleasant side effects.

Exercise is a vital ingredient of life. It helps you to lay firm ground to build a beautiful slim and trim body. Various weight loss exercises for the whole body have been discussed in detail in this book. Besides, it teaches a style of eating and learning to select low-calorie foods. It suggests many ways in which day-to-day eating habits may be modified in the pursuit of slimness and good health.

Pregnancy and menopause are important phases in a woman's life when a lot of care has to be taken to keep the body healthy, youthful and slim. The last chapters contain effective exercises designed to make pregnancy more comfortable, labour and childbirth less painful, and sex life enjoyable with the help of prenatal and post-natal exercise programs illustrated with photographs. Special post-natal exercises and food regimens have been designed to help you get back in shape gradually after childbirth.

—*Parvesh Handa*

Contents

Contents

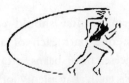

Routine Slimming Programme for Beginners

Tips for beginners

○ Exercises should be done in open air, or in a well-ventilated room.

○ Wear clothes of lightest description – shorts, for preference.

○ Concentration when exercising is very important. Close the eyes and visualise the particular, affected muscle or set of muscles you intend to treat. Do not allow the mind to wander during exercise.

○ You need complete relaxation after exercising.

○ Breathing must be through the nose – on no account should the mouth be used for breathing.

○ All exercise movements must be performed slowly and without jerks.

○ Muscle exercise is important. Particular muscle or set of muscles should be contracted with vigour for a second or two. The process may be repeated until the muscles become slightly tired. Remember, fatigue must be avoided.

○ The best time for exercise is early in the morning before taking a bath.

○ Do not exercise within an hour of a meal.

○ Give the muscles rest for a day in the week.

○ Exercise with the feeling and intention that the body shall benefit.

○ The ideal form of diet should consist of five parts carbohydrates, one part each of albumin (meat, fish, eggs, milk, cheese, peas, beans, etc) and fat (butter, oil, egg-yolk, nuts, etc.). Eat plenty of raw fresh fruit and vegetables in the form of salads.

○ Cook foods preferably in a fireproof glass casserole so as to conserve the vitamins.

○ Fresh food should be preferred to canned, frozen and preserved foods. Use brown sugar instead of white. Don't eat polished rice. Potatoes should be boiled, baked or roasted in their skins.

○ Cod-liver oil is beneficial for growing children involved in regular practice of exercising.

○ Drink a glass of plain cold water after exercise in the morning and about six to eight glasses during the day.

○ Eat either an apple or an orange, or begin breakfast with raw fresh fruit after having a glass of water in the morning.

○ Wear light, breathable underclothing in winter and summer.

○ Avoid tight-fitting clothes or tight-fitting shoes. Do not overload yourself with heavy clothing.

○ Take bath after exercise and before breakfast.

○ A cold shower bath is beneficial. Warm bath should be taken once a week before going to bed.

○ Sun bathing should not be indulged in by those of a nervous temperament or by those suspected to have had tuberculosis, without consulting a doctor. The exposure to sun should not be for more than ten minutes in the beginning. Gradually, increase the duration.

Tips to fight overweight

What makes people overweight?

Overeating is the sole cause for overweight. In other words, total caloric intake exceeds total caloric needs.

How does a glandular disorder cause overweight?

Glandular disorders very rarely cause overweight. The majority of obese people are overweight because they eat more food than they need.

What are the harmful effects of taking a very large quantity of thyroid extract in an attempt to reduce weight?

If excessive quantity of thyroid extract is taken, the metabolic rate may increase beyond normal limits, and the patient may develop a condition similar to hyperthyroidism, which may lead to heart damage.

Should injections be taken for weight reduction?

Some doctors administer injections to help patients reduce weight. These medications usually consist of diuretic drugs and their results are only temporary because they cause water loss rather than loss of weight due to a decrease in fat tissue. There is no permanent weight loss from its use. There is no harmful effect of injections in case of temporary medication. However, if the treatment is continued for a longer period, this may seriously alter the chemical body reactions.

What is the permanent treatment to lose weight?

There are a few medicines to reduce appetite temporarily enabling the patient to take less food, but their effect is seldom long lasting.

What are the medicines to lose appetite?

Most of the drugs belong to the amphetamine group such as Benzedrine, Dexedrine, etc. They often make people less hungry. There are also certain cellulose products that are bulk producers and are supposed to give the patient the sensation that his/her stomach is full. Amphetamines are habit-forming medicines and should be avoided.

11

Is the effect of these medicines harmful?

Both amphetamines and cellulose products can be very harmful and their use should be limited.

What is the role of physical exercise in weight loss?

Exercise plays an important role in weight loss. Short, irregular spurts of activity are ineffective, but regular supervised exercise will definitely produce weight loss.

What is the best way to lose weight?

To eat proper, balanced, medically approved, low-caloric diet.

Should all obese people lose weight?

Seek advice of a doctor. Many people suffering from ulcers or other intestinal upsets should lose weight gradually under close medical supervision.

Is obesity hereditary?

Obesity is often influenced by environment. A child who grows up in a family of heavy eaters is likely to become a heavy eater himself and therefore, will tend to become obese.

Why certain people in the habit of eating huge quantity of food tend to remain thin?

These people may appear to eat tremendously, but actually they eat foods of low caloric value. Also, they are seen to be physically active and burn up more calories.

Sometimes, there are people who eat large quantity of food but lose weight on account of suffering from diabetes and hyperthyroidism.

Why some people fail to lose weight even when they diet strenuously?

Studies reveal that some people do not diet as carefully or take sufficiently low amount of caloric intake as required. It has been found that it is extremely rare for a patient to adhere to a prescribed diet, and usually he fails to lose weight.

Will all overweight people who diet properly lose weight?

Yes, provided their caloric intake is less than their caloric need. If the diet is of low caloric value, it causes weight loss. If the diet is unbalanced, it may cause serious vitamin or protein deficiencies.

Why do women often put on weight at menopause?

There is lesser calorie need in women when they grow older. They need a hundred fewer calories a day for each ten years they advance beyond middle age.

What is the relationship between the length of life span and obesity?

Longevity is decreased in direct proportion to the degree of obesity.

Is there any relationship between emotional state of a person and his/her weight?

Emotionally upset people usually remain under tension, resulting in sometimes overeating and many times under-eating.

What is the relationship between being overweight and coronary heart disease?

Coronary heart disease is seen more among obese people and in those who eat high-fat diet.

What is cholesterol?

It is fatty substance found in certain foods and also in blood. The cholesterol level varies in different people. The body produces its own cholesterol.

What type of fatty foods should be avoided?

Animal fats, because vegetable fats do not seem to cause much harm. Prefer a diet that is composed of two-third part fruit, vegetables, cereals and whole grains. Only one-third of your calories should come from meat and dairy products. Cut the fat. Three principal important dietary factors have an impact on blood cholesterol levels. Saturated fat elevates blood cholesterol. Polyunsaturated fat lowers blood cholesterol. Dietary cholesterol contributes to elevate blood cholesterol to a lesser degree than saturated fat. Saturated fat comprises of meat, butter, cheese and hydrogenated oil. Wherever possible, replace these items with fish, poultry, low-fat dairy products and polyunsaturated oils such as corn, safflower and soya bean.

13

What is the role of exercise to decrease the level of cholesterol in blood?

Exercise decreases the build up of cholesterol blockage inside arteries. Exercise increases the body's ability to clear fat from the blood after meals. Take garlic and onions. Raw garlic can reduce harmful blood fats. Cut back on coffee. Smoking, too, increases cholesterol levels in blood. Tobacco smoking has a tendency to cut one's appetite. It is seen many who stop smoking will reach out for a sweet instead of a cigarette and ultimately start gaining weight.

Should people who are dieting strenuously take vitamin supplements?

They should, if they are on an unbalanced weight-reducing diet. However, a well-balanced, weight-reducing diet will not require the addition of vitamins.

Why do some people become constipated while they are on a weight-reducing diet?

This occasionally happens because the total mass of food intake reduces. Seek medical advice in order to aid bowel evacuation.

Should children as well as adults go on low-calorie diets to lose weight?

It is very important for children to maintain normal weight. If children develop poor eating habits and become obese in childhood, it will be much more difficult for them to stay thin when they mature.

Will it harm the body if there is loss in weight too quickly?

It will be very harmful for health.

What are the harmful effects on obese people as compared to thin people?

Obese people tend to get high blood pressure and diabetes more often. They develop tumours and cancers more frequently as compared to thin people.

Should salt be restricted in weight-reducing diets?

Salt restriction permits a greater loss of fluid and therefore, a greater weight loss. This, however, is a temporary loss.

Does drinking of alcoholic beverages tend to produce obesity?

An average drink contains about a hundred calories and also serves to stimulate appetite.

How it is possible to carry out spot reducing?

All of the advertisements offering losing weight in certain areas of the body are fallacious. There is no efficient method of taking off weight in a particular area of the anatomy.

What are the common causes for being underweight?

These include chronic infections or diseases (such as tuberculosis, kidney ailments and liver disorder, etc.), glandular imbalance (such as excess activity of thyroid gland or malfunctioning of pituitary gland), neurotic manifestations (lack of taste for eating), poor eating habits associated with an irregular lifestyle, excess physical activities and too little sleep.

Do emotions play any part in causing underweight?

People under great emotional strain may eat less and lose weight.

What is the best way to gain weight?

Eat more calories than used. Foods containing higher calories are cream, eggs, carbohydrates, butter, etc. Develop a habit of taking four to five meals a day instead of the usual three. If being underweight has a psychological cause, attempt to eliminate it.

Do vitamin pills help increase weight?

Not if the vitamin intake in the diet is normal.

What are the medications that can aid one to eat more?

There are stimulants that may increase the appetite, but their effectiveness is not very satisfactory.

What type of diet should I choose to become thin?

Eating too little will not make you thin. Ignore all the fad diets and very low-cal diets; these will make you fat and miserable. Don't skip meals – the optimum diet plan is five regular, small meals a day. Make a habit to eat at short intervals in the day and keep dinner as a light snack. Low fat and high fibre is the only way to go. Try to eat foods which derive no more than 20% of their calories from fat. Remember that one gram of fat equals nine calories. You need to follow the healthy eating pyramid guidelines, which recommends that the largest part of your diet (say between 30-45%) should come from whole grains like cereals, brown bread, rice and pasta. Vegetables should form 15-25% of your daily intake, followed by fruits (10-15%). Dairy products and meats should not increase more than 10% each in your diet. Added fats, oils and sweets should not be more than 5%.

What is the best weight-reducing plan?

Slow weight loss is the best. The biggest problem with traditional weight loss diets is the nutritional deficiency which undermines your immune system, promotes diseases and also makes you fat. If your diet lacks vitamins and minerals, your body will want to eat more to make up for the deficiency.

Why do diets make us fat?

Our body has its own set point – a weight at which the body happily settles. Put on weight and it responds by burning energy faster. Lose weight and it burns calories more slowly in an effort to hang on to the set point. Reduce your daily calories level only a little, not more than 20%. The only way not to trigger your body's defence of its set point is to lose about ½ kg to 1 kg a week. When you start that reduction, cut those calories from fat.

What is the fastest way to burn fat?

Strenuous swimming burns four times more calories than strenuous running. Stick to the more energetic form crawl. Sauna bath (steam bath) is equally important to lose weight. 15 minutes of sitting in a sauna equals to 2 km. of running. Consistency is the key to successful fat-burning, so it is essential to choose activities that you enjoy and that fit in with your lifestyle. If aerobic classes leave you cold, choose a form of exercise that suits you – it might be power walking, playing tennis or half-an-hour on a stair-climber. If you intend to join a gym, choose one that is within walking distance of your residence.

What is the difference between hunger and appetite?

Hunger is the body's requirement for food and is influenced by physical needs. Appetite is the desire to eat. That is why one feels hungry on spotting his favourite pastry despite a full stomach. It is because the pastry activates one's appetite. So, controlling appetite will help control obesity.

What is the secret of quick weight loss?

Maintain discipline and regular meal timings. Skipping breakfast and eating cheese sandwiches or oily 'chana-bhatura', followed by heavy lunch with frequent cups of tea and coffee, a few drinks to unwind in the evening, and scrumptious dinner of curry and rice is definitely going to make you bulky and disfigured. Here are few important tips to fight obesity:

O Eat more raw fruits and vegetables.

O Say 'no' to sugar. The body can derive all the sugar it needs from the balanced, nutritious food you eat. The extra sugar does nothing but encourage obesity.

O A regular exercise helps lose weight. The benefits of exercising include: an increase in stamina, stabilised appetite, increased metabolism, improvement in blood circulation and haemoglobin levels.

O Eat small, frequent meals.

Does a woman become fatter with increasing age or after giving birth to children?

As a woman ages above 30, her low levels of activity and hormonal changes cause to lose lean muscle mass. That slows her metabolic rate, so it burns food less efficiently. On exercising, we burn lesser because of lean muscle mass. A study reveals that childbearing results in permanent weight gain. According to information, after the pregnancies, women gain 2-3 kg – the more the children, the greater the gain. However, during pregnancy, women on average gain 13 kg – 3 kg of which is the baby, the rest being fluid, placenta (a tube feeding the baby in womb) and fat stored to produce milk. Breastfeeding is one of the ways to regain the pre-pregnancy figure because it helps use up the stored fat of pregnancy.

Do the sexes gain weight differently?

Women tend to gain weight usually around their hips and thighs, whereas men put it on around their stomachs. However, according to a study, hormonal changes during menopause tend to cause a shift of weight from hips to the belly. Men whose waists are more than 100 cm and women who measure more than 90 cm should take it as a warning sign. It is seen, women in all age groups diet more than men – between 20-40% more.

What are the dangers of being overweight?

That depends on how fat you are. The real danger is obesity when you are 20% above the ideal body weight. The risks due to obesity include suffering from diabetes, high blood pressure, high cholesterol, indigestion, heart disease, gall bladder diseases and some forms of cancer.

What to do if one regains lost weight?

90% of dieters usually regain their weight. Remember, diet alone won't do because it depletes the lean muscle that is so effective in burning fat. Exercise alone may not do it either because it reduces fat, not extra weight. However, diet along with exercise may help control obesity to some extent.

What is the role of exercise and anti-cellulite cream in fighting obesity?

Exercise burns calories, increases metabolism and replaces fat with muscle. But exercise as much as it takes to make you feel good. Body firming and contouring creams and gels help to make skin smooth but they cannot melt away fat. Remember, cellulite is a quack term for ordinary fat, which cannot be spot-reduced. Cellulite looks like a fat cell.

How to detox body to slim down?

The present 21st century lifestyle places high demand on your body beauty. Make sure to regularly deep cleanse your skin and hair to eliminate toxins. Massage, brushing and bathing are prominent ways to detox your body and slim down.

○ *Massage* improves circulation and lymph drainage, and helps banish cellulite. Aromatherapy experts advise mixing up your own blend with 10 ml of carrier oil (such as sweet almond oil) and a few drops of pure essential oil (such as lemon, juniper or grapefruit) designed to stimulate and purify. Massage concentrate gently once a day on problem areas such as your thighs, buttocks and abdomen as long as it takes for the oil to be absorbed. Remember, this is not your spa-type massage – it's carried out for circulation, applied after a bath while the skin is damp and warm.

○ *Body brushing* is good for busting cellulite besides getting a smooth and firm skin. Choose a brush with natural firm bristles and long handle. Brush up for about five minutes on back, arms, legs and tummy towards your heart in a circular, clockwise movement in the morning before you shower. Start off slowly and gently in the beginning and then after about a week be more vigorous when your skin gets used to the pressure.

○ *Bathing* is good for easing tension. Add to the water Epsom salts to help your skin to eliminate toxins besides melting away fat. Avoid using soap. Aromatherapy oils, sea salt, mud or algae help to stimulate. Fill the tub up to your neck and wallow in it for 15 minutes concentrating on breathing deeply, not more than twice a week. Remember not to over-stimulate your body.

19

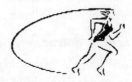

Chapter-2

Programme to Treat Obesity

A surplus fat by 10 – 15% over normal weight must be considered as overweight. Beyond that it is obesity. Over 30% above the normal weight is extreme obesity. Overweight not only affects your looks, but also your health. Beware of overweight, which causes various troubles as mentioned below:

1. Circulation troubles such as palpitation, pain in the heart, heart trouble, high blood pressure, diabetes, gout.

2. Psychological and Nervous Troubles.

3. Digestive disorders such as dilation of stomach, painful digestion, inflammation and spasms of the intestines and congestion of the liver.

4. Genital disorders, because the infiltration of fat into the nervous and glandular tissues controls sexual appetite and can cause temporary impotence. If timely care is taken to slim the body, the sexual desire will return.

Chart of average weight and measurements (in inches)

Height	60	61	62	63	64	65	66	67	68	70
Weight (kg)	49	51	52	55	56	58	59	60	60	62
Bust	32	32.5	33	33.5	34	34.5	35	35.5	36	36.5
Waist	22.5	23	23.5	24	24.5	25	25.5	26	26.5	27
Hips	33	33.5	34	34.5	35	35.5	36	36.5	37	38
Neck	12.5	12.5	13	13	13.5	13.5	14	14	14.5	14.5
Arm	10	10.5	10.5	11	11	11.5	11.5	12	12	12.5
Thigh	18.5	18.5	19	19.5	20	20	20.5	21	21	21.5
Calf	12.5	13	13	13	13.5	14	14	14	14.5	15
Wrist	6	6	6	6.5	7	7	7	7.5	8	8
Ankle	7	7	7.5	8	8	8.5	8.5	9	9	10

What is overweight

Overweight is the symptom of fundamental imbalances in your body, emotions and mind. These imbalances include the following:

○ Emotional imbalance.

○ Nutritional imbalance.

○ Physical imbalance.

○ Mental imbalance.

The best health professional helping you lose weight is a person who understands and can help solve the various nutritional, metabolic, hormonal, immune and lifestyle problems that actually cause overweight. The practitioner should be able to medically investigate and correct each of the following factors in weight problems:

○ Depleted brain chemistry.

○ A low-calorie diet, which is a common cause of overeating.

○ Blood sugar problems, including medical problems such as hypoglycemia, diabetes, and exhaustion of adrenal glands.

○ Low thyroid function.

○ Food allergies and addictions.

○ Hormonal imbalances as stated above.

○ Yeast overgrowth with candida, which causes carbohydrate craving.

○ A deficiency of essential fatty acids.

What is fatty overweight

Fatty overweight is usually seen in men where the increase in weight is spread uniformly over the whole body. It is more often noticeable over the upper half portion of the body, particularly on head, neck, arms and trunk. There is both an excess of fat and over-development of muscles. It is also called energetic overweight, and harmful effects include cholesterol, gout, stones, hypertension, coronary thrombosis, diabetes, etc. The main causes of fatty overweight are the following:

1. *Heredity factor:* There is family tendency to stoutness, which is more often the inheritance of the habit of overeating rather than a truly genetic factor.

2. *The age factor:* When some people eat excessively up to a certain age and the obesity occurs due to poor functioning of the system.

3. *Due to overeating:* As a result of taking in too many calories with food, and building up a reserve in the form of an overdeveloped layer of fat.

4. *Sedentary life:* Not only because of absorbing too much, but also because of using relatively too little calories and not taking enough muscular exercise.

5. Part played by nervous factors.

6. *The effect of your glands:* When the fatty overweight is accompanied by glandular symptoms which usually disappear when the obesity is cured. Over-secretion of sub-renal glands play a major role.

How to treat fatty overweight

Necessary steps should be taken to reduce intake of food and combat extra amount of fat. The following treatments are helpful to reduce obesity:

Dieting: Is the most essential part of the treatment. There is need of lesser quantity but a quality diet. Lower the number of calories taken daily (between 1300 to 1600 calories every 24 hours). Cut down fat and carbohydrates to a minimum, but retain a sufficient amount of protein.

Food you may eat

○ Non-fatty soups, vegetable broths without bread, slightly salted.

○ Mutton, lean fish, lean poultry – without sauce or butter.

22

- Egg (one a day).
- Small quantities of fresh butter and liquid paraffin.
- Fresh or condensed milk (skimmed and unsweetened).
- Fresh cheese with low fat content.
- Potatoes in very small quantity.
- All green vegetables and fruits.
- Salt in very small quantity.
- Fruit juices, herbal teas and light wines. Never drink when you are eating.

Food you must not eat
- Bread, biscuits, pastries.
- Fatty soups, fat meats and fatty fish.
- Meat in sauces and stews.
- Fat pork meats.
- Fried foods.
- Lard, margarine, butter, oil, cream and milk products.
- Cornflakes, starch, flour and rice.
- Fatty, fermented and salted cheese.
- Dried vegetables and mushrooms.
- Bananas, chestnuts, walnuts, jam, syrup, honey, cocoa and chocolate.
- Wine, beer, cider and all kinds of alcoholic or sweetened drinks.

Exercises and Gymnastics
- *Take energetic exercises:* Physical training, gymnastics, exercises and sports of all kinds. If you are too obese, you must consult the doctor or an expert for suitable exercises.
- Gentle activities, including walking, help to reduce extra weight.

Eliminate excess water: By sucking out a large amount of water in order to eliminate it by drugs that cause water to be absorbed into the intestines, by use of diuretics, sudation, and sweating.

Use of drugs: Hunger can be minimised by the use of drugs. But these drugs should not to be used when the patient is not a big eater or if he/she can control appetite without too much difficulty. These appetite-reducing drugs (psychamines) are available in pill form. These drugs may cause fewer secondary complications such as insomnia and palpitation. These drugs, like many others, if taken uninterruptedly, prove habit-forming. You may avoid this by going without them for ten days every month and relying on your will power during that time. Gradually, you will rid of these drugs. Your doctor will take advantage of this pause to increase your urinary output by means of diuretic drugs. Heart patients and pregnant women must avoid taking such harmful drugs.

Psychological treatment: Remember, emotional shock can be a cause of overweight. This must be fought by personal determination. However, psychamine drugs to reduce appetite can be of great assistance. But consult a doctor before taking such drugs. Consult a doctor in case you are unable to control the disorder.

Hydro-thermal treatment: This is recommended as a useful auxiliary means of getting rid of superfluous weight.

You are fat-prone, if you:

1. Like to eat very well or eat much.
2. Have sedentary habits or a sedentary job.
3. You put on weight during holidays.
4. Are emotionally upset and worry makes you lose weight.
5. Massage and douches have little effect.
6. Sweat session is moderate but there is lasting loss of weight.

7. Are cutting down on your food, which has a noticeable effect.

8. Overweight has overtaken you at a time other than at a stage of sexual development, such as puberty, menopause, pregnancy, etc.

9. Are affected by overweight at the upper part of body, such as arms, shoulders and face as much as or more than the lower part.

10. Are overweight, accompanied by circulation trouble.

11. Rarely feel cold.

Some do's

○ Weigh yourself every 28 days.

○ Cut down on your food, and cut out, in particular, biscuits, bread, cakes.

○ Use little salt but no sugar.

○ Breakfast on tea and apples.

○ Don't drink while you are eating.

○ If necessary, reduce your appetite by taking psychamines an hour before taking meals.

○ Take Foam Bath or Turkish Bath.

○ Have 20 minutes of physical exercises preceded by muscular limbering up, every morning; and energetic sports.

○ Drink diuretic fluids.

Some don'ts

○ Weigh yourself very frequently.

○ Lose patience.

○ Let yourself become constipated and take drugs of your own accord without consulting a doctor.

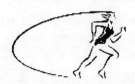

Chapter-3

Programme to Fight Watery Overweight

Watery overweight is the commonest form of female overweight described as spongy obesity. The main characteristic of this type of overweight is that it is paradoxical.

Symptoms: This type of overweight occurs almost solely in women, mostly in young women and teenage girls just entering the early years of adulthood. It may also occur at the menopause stage after the age of 50. Watery overweight usually affects the upper limbs and predominates over the lower half of the body – generally on the hips and the buttocks. From there the overweight extends to the stomach, the thighs and the inside of the knees. The patient complains of cold feet, hands, and chilblains occur even in summer with red and damp appearance. Moreover, red blotches appear on the legs, which increase in size, become rough, coarse-grained, veined, stiff, and hurt when touched. The patient often complains of a frequently twisted ankle. The nails break or split. In nearly all cases of watery overweight, irregular and painful periods among women, intestinal swelling, a painful tension in the chest and nervousness are the common symptoms. The periods last two or three days and are usually accompanied by frequent headaches.

Causes of watery overweight

1. *Food:* Dieting is an important part of the treatment. Overeating does not usually account for overweight. The lack of balance in feeding with too much water (not

enough albumin) leads to stopping of the normal chemical reactions through its alkalising character, and prevents the body from getting rid of the surplus water, which starts accumulating in the tissues.

2. *Salt:* Plays a significant part and holds water. When menstruation starts, the blood becomes loaded with salt, with retention of water during periods. In order to combat the retention of water and thirst, we must strictly limit the intake of salt.

3. *Exercise:* Plays an important part. Heavy exercises generally cause to put on extra weight, whereas rest and lying down reduces weight considerably.

4. *Age:* It is very important. Paradoxical overweight occurs at the time of sexual development and change. A woman can expect an improvement with marriage and her first pregnancy. At the menopause, a woman can expect her circulatory condition to become stable.

5. *Endocrine factors:* It is a matter of phases of sexual development rather than age in female sex. Retention of water in the tissues of body owing to decrease in urinary elimination is encouraged not only by lack of balance in food intake, but also by ovarian or pituitary activity. Normally, women gain a little weight (about 500 gm.) when their period starts, which becomes normal when it is over. In case of watery overweight, this loss doesn't occur and a woman puts on weight successively at every monthly period. Estrogenic hormones cause weight gain in women, and induce abnormal retention of water. Watery overweight often occurs at a stage of sexual development such as puberty, pregnancy, miscarriage, a natural or induced menopause.

6. *Psychological factors:* The emotional elements can often effect severe mental shock.

7. *The electro-chemical balance of the body fluids:* Keeps balance of the blood and the resulting lymphatic fluids. In case of watery overweight, a deficiency of metallic catalytic

27

agents such as zinc, copper, nickel, manganese or perhaps cobalt is observed (varying from one patient to another). Treatment by administering small doses of these metals as per recommendation of your doctor results in favourable changes in the electrical charges of the different elements in the blood, thereby preventing certain abnormal chemical activities.

Treatment

Diet

Unbalanced eating is in the major cause of watery overweight. Dieting is the leading factor in its treatment Observe the following precautions:

1. Never drink water (or any liquid) with your meals. Drink very little between meals, if required.
2. Don't salt your food.
3. Eat few vegetables and plenty of meats in case of non-vegetarians.
4. No watery foods, such as soup, juicy fruits, melon, etc.
5. Consult a doctor or a dietician before embarking on strict diets.

Rest

Exercise, overwork, walking, fatigue and late nights encourage overweight. You must relax and rest. Good results are achieved from resting in bed. A lying down position causes an increase in urination. Cases are known of young women regularly losing 5 to 7 kg a week during three weeks in bed.

Massage

Reflex therapeutic massage acts indirectly by its effect on nervous system and brings a relaxing effect.

Sweating, laxatives and diuretics

Paradoxically, these are ineffective in cases of watery overweight. They cannot bring about a permanent weight loss, as there is no surplus fat to break down. That is why sweating, laxatives and diuretics are of no use. The only solution is to gradually reduce the abnormal need of the tissues for water by cutting down water intake over a long period and by diminishing the intake of salt, and by taking on the electro-chemical balance of the blood.

You have watery overweight, if:

- ○ You eat moderately. Putting yourself on a vegetable and fruit diet; even cut down your food considerably.
- ○ You overstrain yourself physically and mentally.
- ○ Rest and relaxation are immediately beneficial.
- ○ Emotions and worry cause you to put on weight.
- ○ You don't feel really well.
- ○ Sweating causes temporary loss of weight.
- ○ You have serious trouble with your periods, which sometimes diminish or disappear altogether.
- ○ The overweight occurs at the time of change in sexual development.
- ○ The overweight is predominantly in the lower part of the body, on hips, buttocks and thighs.
- ○ You have serious circulation troubles when legs become veined, dry and rough, and the ankles are heavy and swollen by the evening.
- ○ You have chilblains every winter.
- ○ Your nails split.

What to do in case of watery overweight

- ○ Weigh yourself every 28 days.
- ○ Do not eat bread and cakes. Avoid vegetables, juicy fruits and soups. Eat eggs, meat and cheese (unsalted).
- ○ For breakfast, preferably eat an egg, cheese or yogurt.
- ○ Don't eat and drink at the same time. Drink very little between meals.

○ Rest and relax as much as possible.

○ Drink mineral waters, which encourage total elimination.

What you must avoid in case of watery overweight

○ Weigh yourself constantly.

○ Lose patience.

○ Go without food, or cut out meat and put yourself on vegetables and fruits.

○ Indulge in physical exercise and exhausting sports.

○ Go to bed late.

○ Take strong purgatives.

○ Get constipated.

○ Take drugs without medical supervision.

○ Follow a dry diet without medical supervision.

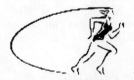

Chapter-4

Programme to Beat Cellulite

The difference between cellulite and fatty obesity or watery overweight is that it affects certain limited areas on body, not the large areas on the body. A woman with cellulite may have it only on the hips or the nape of her neck, or in both legs. The rest of the body remains unaffected. Beauty consultants believe that certain herbal formulas and natural ways have restorative powers that can help smooth skin affected by cellulite. Fragrant herbal plant oils frequently used for massage (generally called aromatherapy) are absorbed directly through the skin and combat cellulite. These aromatherapy oils are readily available in health food stores.

What is cellulite

Cellulite is an inflammation of the connective tissue caused by poisons accumulating there instead of being thrown out by the body. The most common of these poisons are uric and oxalic acids. In case of cellulite, the double chin, thick shoulders and swollen ankles are stuffed with organic waste matter, which is normally rejected through urine, sweat and bowels. This waste matter often collects in the connective tissue. The connective tissue is to be found in the body wherever there are no organs. Under the skin, it is known as subcutaneous cellular tissue. In case of cellulite, this connective tissue fills with lymph containing much waste matter, which irritates it and causes it to contract. It then fills with water. Water thickens into mucus, which in turn becomes semi-solid matter. This congests the cellular tissue, which then becomes painful. This is cellulite. Cellulite is not exclusive to women. Nearly 30% of cases afflict men. Most women have disfiguring cellulite – loose flabby fat trapped in hardened networks of elastin and collagen fibres. There is no miracle cure for it. However, you can see great results by effective natural ways.

How to diagnose cellulite

As described above, when suffering from cellulite there is an accumulation of loose flabby fat with fluid and toxins trapped into hardened deeper levels of the skin. Cellulite begins on the inside surface of the thighs and knees, covering up the bone projections. It quickly moves down to thicken ankles, which disappear from view. This thickening becomes more and more pronounced and soon affects the whole leg from the ankle to the knee. Gradually but relentlessly, over the months and years, the thickening of lower limbs continues and the sides of the thighs swell out in their turn. The hips become heavy with rolls of fat and affect the buttocks and rest of the body, which include the thick neck, swollen napes and heavy shoulders, thighs, hips, bottom and even tummy. To check cellulite, just do this simple test. Squeeze the skin of your upper thigh between the thumb and index finger. If the flesh feels lumpy and looks bumpy, then you suffer from cellulite.

At first the tissues have a soft consistency and are not painful. Sometimes it is difficult to distinguish from watery or fatty infiltration. Later, pinching the skin is painful and may produce small wrinkles. Cellulite may be suspected from the badly nourished appearance of the skin – rough, greyish and cold. At the stage of confirmed cellulite, the symptoms are clear when the skin gives a feeling of padding. The skin adheres to the underlying tissues instead of making for suppleness, and becomes inflamed. The pinching is usually painful and causes bruising. At the atrophy stage, you will feel underneath the skin small balls or little grains: a kind of nodule, which rolls around under your fingers. The organs attacked by cellulite include the inside surface of the thighs, knees, ankles, hips, nape of the neck, back of arms, shoulder blades, spinal column, on the forehead and lower part of the face. Cellulite overweight does not bring the organic disorders caused by obesity. One can die from obesity but not of cellulite. More serious cellulite will give rise to nervous pressure resulting in severe pains, which occur more often at night giving rise to insomnia that contributes to the disorder of the nervous system.

Factors causing cellulite and the treatment

Cellulite is caused and aggravated by the following:

○ A poor diet of low-fibre, high fat food, which puts great pressure on the body's digestive system to expel toxins.

○ Lack of exercise and stress often slow down blood circulation and the lymphatic system.

○ Hereditary factor.

Heredity, feeding (a cellulite mother often has a cellulite daughter), abnormal activity of the liver, generally due to dieting and sedentariness are some of the other factors favouring cellulite. To burn up toxins in the body, exercise your muscles. Toxins can be burnt up only by oxygen. Oxygen can consume poisons at only two points: the lungs and the muscles, which work together for purification in the body. Fatigue, like sedentariness, is an important factor in cellulite and these can be relieved by regular exercising, but avoid over-exerting your body. Learn to breathe in open air. Avoid toxic foods and alcohol that attacks three basic defenses – the digestive system, the nervous system and the kidney system. For the treatment of cellulite, following steps are advised:

Dieting

Eat judiciously with low calorie content. Good food should make up for the normal wear and tear. Ban everything which is highly seasoned – condiments, spices, salt, pepper or toxic substances such as coffee, tea, alcohol, tobacco, highly fermented cheese or too acid – tomatoes, lemons, and over-cooked foods such as stews, fatty pork meats, sauces, cooked butter, fried foods. A cellulite should avoid as much as possible oily fish, some of the vegetables (broad beans, split peas, soya), all dry fruits, milk products, tobacco, all confectionery, all spicy things (mustard, pickles, garlic) and drinks. Eat meals at regular hours (do not eat between meals). Try hard to eat in peace, away from noise and be completely relaxed during meals. A cellulite will need only a cooling diet, rich in green vegetables and well-balanced menus.

Exercise

Physical exercise plays a part in burning up poisons. So if you are going to stop the body fluids becoming clogged, make sure that you exercise your muscles sufficiently. But too violent exercise resulting in fatigue and stress increases the poisons in the system. Cellulites need plenty of fresh air (open air walking) and active muscular life. There is no single rule for how long you should walk or have exercise – each has his own staying power and resistance. The length of walk or exercise may be increased from five minutes the first day to half-an-hour after a week, 45 minutes after a fortnight, half an hour twice a day after three weeks. Do not wear high-heeled shoes.

Rest

It is not only immoderate physical exercise that causes strain, everyday life (the harassed life) causes it too. Remember, the body substances and nerve centres have to be restored at regular intervals and need periodic rest. If your working life is already exhausting, don't add extra strain to it. Generally speaking, eight hours' sleep is essential for people who use up a lot of energy. The ideal is to go to bed at 10 p.m. and get up at 6 a.m.

Breathing

Breathing is equally important in burning up the poisons in the blood as oxygen is the great purifier of the bloodstream. Lungs, too, need all the vital forces in the atmosphere, which come from the sun, from the earth and are breathed out by every living thing, such as flowers, birds and trees. We must find fresh air. We must shun stuffy atmospheres and crowded streets as much as possible because of our need for this vital force. Start breathing in gently, first inflating the upper part of the thorax, and moving arms to the horizontal position and then slightly backwards. The complete breathing in process should take 6 to 12 seconds. Breathing out should be done slowly. Begin by collapsing the upper part of the chest, then the lower part, and end by contracting the stomach. To empty the chest completely, lower the arms, the shoulders and the head bent slightly forward and back slightly arched.

Massage

Gentle and gradually increasing massage, which arouses sensation rather than pain, always dispels cellulite from the place to which it is applied. Various massage movements applied on the body will be described in detail in one of the coming chapters. Remember, massage should never cause pain, but should be hard enough all the same to arouse more sensitivity than it would have done on a perfectly healthy area.

The best time for massage is in the morning, when the inflammation of the cellulite tissue is at its minimum. Cellulite is always more evident in the evening because of fatigue. Morning massage can be deeper, hence more effective. Do the massage three times a week, about 35 minutes each time, having draining for 5 minutes, roll-massage for 5 minutes, rapid massage on all the least affected areas for 10 minutes, direct massage on most painful areas for 10 minutes and general draining movements for 5 minutes. Finish with a cold shower and friction with a loofah or a rough towel. You will be able to recognise good and effective massage by the fact that the ganglions (of the groins for the legs, of the armpits for the arms) have enlarged and do not hurt after the session. If the massage is too violent, the ganglions will not enlarge until the next day and will be painful.

Boosting your circulation

Use exfoliating loofahs to boost circulation and lymphatic system. Exfoliation can be done with a body brush or a hand mitt in long sweeping movements on the affected area, working in the direction of the heart for 3-5 minutes. Loofah dissolves cellulite.

To make loofah scrub: Mix 1-2 drops each of lemon oil and fennel seed oil in a vegetable scrub (which contains papain enzymes). Make a paste by adding water, rub with soft brush gently to avoid scraping your skin.

Burning cellulite with lipostim

Lipostim calorie burner pads are smeared with slimming oil and placed on strategic areas of the body which contain stubborn cellulite. Unwanted layers of fat are burned off by pulsar mode in this 30-minute procedure, followed by massage with slimming oil for about 10 minutes to tone up the sluggish muscles and tissues. Loose and flabby skin is tightened with warm aromatic steam containing juniper berry oil (available at a herbal store). This process helps to get rid of 50-60% cellulite fat.

Follow a detox diet

The detox diet works well to flush out toxins and gives a healthy surge of vital energy to the body. A 5-day detox programme is described below. During the course of this programme you can drink unlimited quantities of warm water. But avoid drinking cold water, tea, coffee, alcohol and sugar. A daily 30-minute brisk walk is a must to keep muscles fit and fine.

Detox diet programme

○ *Day 1:* Take only coconut water, lime water, wheat water, barley water, tomato juice and 2 teaspoons honey throughout the day.

○ *Day 2:* Take 6 ripe bananas, 4 apples, 200 gm papaya, 10 soaked raisins, 5 prunes (alubukhara), 2 amlas and 6 walnuts during the day.

○ *Day 3:* Take 150 gm raw paneer, cucumber, tomato, boiled moong sprouts, coconut water and 100 ml carrot juice during the day.

○ *Day 4:* Take 6 chapaties or 6 slices of oil-free brown bread, 15 gm white butter, 2 apples, 4 bananas and coconut water during the day.

○ *Day 5:* Take 150 gm boiled white rice, 100 gm moong dal, 100 ml raw tomato juice, 2 bananas and 150 ml pineapple juice during the day.

Night care

Aromatherapy massage works wonders. To prepare massage cream: Mix 2 drops fennel seed oil, 2 drops rosemary oil, 4 drops lemon oil with 2 teaspoons vitamin E cream (400 IU). Massage and leave on cellulite areas at night. Repeat daily for two weeks.

You are suffering from cellulite, if:

1. It is localised and begins on the inside surface of the thighs and knees.
2. The skin is infiltrated, padded and has the elastic consistency.
3. The skin cannot be squeezed and develops the "orange peel" look.
4. The skin hurts when touched.
5. Bruises appear very easily.

What to do in case of cellulite

○ Take regular, well-balanced meals with low calorie content.

○ A daily exercise is recommended but it should not be too energetic. Open-air walking and light sports are very beneficial.

○ Rest as often as possible; relax.

○ Breathe efficiently, with your chest and your stomach.

○ Massage yourself correctly without causing pain or discomfort.

○ Increase the intensity of the massage progressively, but never let it become painful.

○ Before and after massage, do the drainage movement in the direction of lymphatic circulation.

What you must never do

1. Perform intensive physical exercise.
2. Start massaging vigorously right away, thereby causing discomfort.
3. Get bruised after massage.
4. Get tired and stiff after walking.
5. Eat indigestible foods.
6. Drink alcoholic drinks.
7. Indulge in smoking.
8. Drink too much coffee or tea.
9. Live in stuffy atmosphere.
10. Exhaust your nerves too much.
11. Regularly frequent badly ventilated and smoky public places.

Tips to fight obesity

Obesity and overweight complaints are quite common. There are several causes for obesity; majority of them are due to overeating and lack of exercise. The logical way to lose weight is to cut down excess/junk food intake by 100% without affecting the nutritive value of the food consumed, and exercise regularly to burn the extra fat.

1 kg of body fat contains 7500 kcal energy. If you reduce 250 kcal from regular food intake and burn another 250 kcal by exercise – the total calorie reduction amounts to 500 kcal or roughly 3500 kcal per week. Thus the total reduction in weight per month will be 2 kg per month. This is considered to be the safe method of losing weight. All weight watchers should keep in mind the following tips to lose weight till desired limit is reached and to maintain thereafter:

1. Fast for longer periods (10 to 12 days under the supervision of an expert).

2. Reduce butter, fat, fried foods, cheese, cream, soups, sweets and sugar.

3. Avoid cakes, pastries, biscuits and salted nuts. Use only skimmed milk.

4. Stop taking alcohol. Eat more watery vegetables and fruits to satiate the appetite.

5. Do not eat without knowing the caloric value of the food.

Natural ways to fight cellulite

Since cellulite is fat, excess weight can contribute to it. According to Dr. D.S.Jaspal, President of Indian Medical Association (Haryana), eat plenty of fresh fruit and vegetables – low in calories yet packed with nutrients. And drink fruit and vegetable juices. He advises to eat a healthy, balanced diet and get back in balance by resting well. Add about two cups of sea salt to warm bath water and luxuriate in the soothing water for about 15 minutes; this leaves your skin feeling smooth. Here are a few natural ways to reduce cellulite:

○ Combat constipation: People who are constipated on a regular basis usually have cellulite. Eat plenty of high-fibre foods like green vegetables and grains every day.

○ Improve eating habits: Chew your food thoroughly and forgo late night snacks. Drink beverages at room temperature rather than ice-cold. Ice constricts your esophagus and stomach, hindering the flow of digestive enzymes into your stomach.

○ Correct waste-removal system of body: The following techniques will open up the blood vessels in and just below your skin and keep your waste-removal system working properly.

1. Drink at least six to eight glasses of bottled water (distilled or mineral) daily.

2. Salt contributes to water retention and adds to cellulite problems.

3. Kick the coffee and cigarette habits.

4. Dry-brush your skin. It helps improve your circulation. Press a soft-bristled brush gently onto your skin and rotate it in circular movements from head to toe or on cellulite-affected areas.

○ Take up muscle-toning exercises. Work out with weights, which help to fill out the tissue in cellulite-problem areas.

○ Kneading massage: This massage movement on trouble spots, usually in the areas like your thighs and the insides of your knees, helps a lot.

○ Take deep breaths: The oxygen helps burn fat. Deep breaths help clean out toxic carbon dioxide from body cells.

○ Stay calm. Cellulite builds up when the body muscles get tense and stressed. Practice Yoga to fight stress. It teaches you to breathe deeply and give body muscles a good stretch and relaxation.

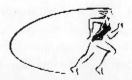

Chapter-5

Essential Supplements for Fat Burning Programme

If you are overweight

There are five categories of weight:

Underweight, Healthy, Overweight, Obese and Very Obese. If you think you are overweight – then see how much? Refer the chart in this book recommending the correct weight according to your height. Always weigh yourself on a reliable scale. Maybe you are within the healthy weight range for your height but still feel flabby. In that case, get to muscle tone to trim on exercise. But if you find yourself overweight then it is time to do something about it. However, a few simple changes in your lifestyle can create a new sense of well-being and the figure required to go with it. First look at the reasons for the extra weight you are carrying. How do you become overweight? There are many reasons for obesity. You may be overweight because of genetic or hormonal reasons. Better you should consult a doctor. Many experts believe that fat people have relatively slow metabolism and their bodies burn energy at a much lower rate than leaner people of the same weight. Other experts suggest overeating is the real problem, while a few blame lack of exercise.

The energy we get from food is used for body's functions and physical activities. The amount of energy varies from person to person. A labourer undergoing hard work might require up to 3500 calories a day, whereas a person on a sitting job needs less than 2000. About two-thirds of these calories are used to maintain body's functioning and provide energy to the organs such as heart, lungs, brain, liver and kidneys, for digestion, growth and maintaining body temperature. The amount of energy spent to keep body well maintained is known as the Basal Metabolic Rate (BMR). Some people burn energy more quickly than others, which depends upon an individual. A person becomes overweight when he eats more than he needs to maintain BMR. The excess energy intake is mainly stored as fat. There are people who seem to eat huge amounts of food and stay slim. Sometimes, the hearty eaters with higher BMR are seen to be much leaner than the people with lower BMR. The digestion process itself requires 10% of the calories consumed. For many people, the weight problem starts in childhood. The overweight can be avoided by having control over eating. Many nutritionists suggest that convenience, i.e. fast foods are much to blame. Processed foods often lack nourishment.

Do I really need exercise

For a beginner, the sudden extra load on the body could be dangerous, especially if he or she is substantially overweight. Find a type of exercise in consultation with your doctor or a health club that can be a part of your life, not just a get-slim-quick type of punishment for your body but to enjoy and shed those extra kilos. Swimming, cycling, brisk walking and playing tennis or badminton are excellent forms of exercise. Unfortunately, in today's fast life, majority of people can make time to watch a regular TV programme or go to the pub to have a few sips but have no time to play sports, or exercise.

Start with a few simple exercises like sit-ups, stretches and climbing stairs in the beginning and gradually build up to fitness. Make it a habit to park the car away from the shopping centre and walk the rest of the way. If you go by bus, get off at an earlier stop and walk up to the destination. If you are working in an office, take the stairs to the upper floors instead of the lift. Remember, every bit of extra activity burns energy and boosts your BMR. The extra energy eventually comes from your reserves of fat.

By exercising regularly one becomes physically fit. Exercise has a balancing effect on stress and anxiety. One feels relaxed when mind and body are occupied with physical activity. When doing vigorous exercise, powerful chemicals called endorphins are released by brain, which act on the body in producing a mental state. Those involved in regular exercise usually sleep more soundly, experience less aches and pains, feel generally calmer and have smaller appetites. So with the right attitude to diet and exercise you really can set yourself on a slimmer, healthier and happier course for life.

If you are seriously overweight, have suffered recent illness, suffer from joint problems or have crossed the age of 40, check with your doctor before you begin. Keep in mind the following cautions:

○ Start exercising slowly and build up gradually.

○ Don't push yourself to exhaustion.

○ Make yourself breathless, not speechless.

○ Warm up and gently stretch before exercising.

○ Don't stop exercise suddenly. Slow the pace to a comfortable level in the end of the your session.

○ Don't exercise after eating a meal, wait at least for an hour or two.

○ Don't ignore when you feel pain in your body.

Tips to look good

○ Avoid saturated fat. Keep intake of fat to a minimum.

○ Avoid refined sugar as much as possible.

○ Keep up intake of dietary fibre.

○ Use fresh, unprocessed, ingredients as much as possible.

○ Try to stick to three meals a day.

○ Eat slowly and chew thoroughly.

○ Avoid over-eating, but at the same time don't starve yourself.

○ Maintain the recommended level of exercise, including activities.

○ Drink plenty of water and fruit juice to keep your appetite under control and 'flush out' bodily wastes and toxins.

○ Enjoy your meal sitting at the table.

○ Don't rush around or watch TV while eating.

○ Adopt healthier habits that promise a slimmer figure and vitality.

A holistic approach—key to overcome overweight

According to a renowned acupuncturist, overweight is the symptom of fundamental imbalances in your body, emotions and mind, which include:

○ Emotional Imbalance in which food is used as a substitute for love affairs and your uncomfortable feelings.

○ Nutritional Imbalance in which the body lacks nutrients for proper functioning of the body.

○ Physical Imbalance due to toxins in the digestive tract that drain your energy and cause you to eat 'stimulating' foods including sugar.

○ Mental Imbalance due to thoughts, which makes you never mindful of what you are eating.

Here are some of the tested methods for correcting the imbalances that are the underlying cause of overweight:

FOOD – that stop cravings

A drink for breakfast is the most important balance-restoring step. This drink is an infusion of essential vitamins, minerals, fatty acids, protein and fibre which helps to cut down on your food cravings as well as depression, irritability, anxiety and many other emotional and mental problems. To prepare it, blend and mix the ingredients such as 1 cup each rice milk, soya milk, apple juice, orange or other fruit juice, 1 banana, 4 fresh strawberries, 1 teaspoon blackstrap molasses, 1 table-spoon each aloe-vera juice, black cherry juice concentrate, powdered green formulations, powdered brewer's or nutritional yeast, raw organic bee pollen (loose) and flaxseed oil.

AFFIRMATIONS - *the right food choices*
Make the right, healthy balanced food choices. Choose one or two affirmations from the following:

- Reveal a clear, healthier, happier in you.
- Think control in yourself.
- Take responsibility of your physical self, wellness and your health.
- Eat to nourish your mind, body and spirit.

REBOUNDING - *the best weight-loss exercise*
Jumping is a good exercise for those trying to lose weight, which helps strengthen the lymphatic system, drains toxins from the body and supports stronger immunity. Exercise for 10 to 20 minutes three to five times a week.

GLUTAMINE - *balance blood sugar, stop cravings*
Food cravings, particularly for sweets and starches, are often caused by low blood sugar or hypoglycemia. Stabilise the delivery of blood sugar to your brain and stop the cravings. Take in consultation with your doctor.

TYROSINE - *for low energy and poor concentration*
When you feel fatigued and brain-fogged, take coffee, cigarettes and sweets to give you a lift. Doctors usually recommend 500 to 2000 mg of tyrosine three times day to make you will feel energised and alert. Always consult a doctor for correct treatment and accurate dosage.

D-PHENYLALANINE - *to overcome emotional pain*
Amino acid d-phenylalanine builds up your brain's reservoir of endorphins and helps to create feelings of pleasure and reduce physical pain. Plenty of high-protein foods are recommended.

GABA - *for stress and tension*

When the muscles are chronically tense, make you feel stressed and burned out, you need relaxation and calmness. You need gamma amino-butyric acid (GABA). GABA taken in combination with glycerine can be even more calming. Better consult your doctor for the treatment.

5-HTP - *for depression, anxiety or low self-esteem*

In case of low levels of the brain chemical serotonin, you will face many emotional and mental problems compelling you to overeat sweets, starches and chocolate causing depression, anxiety, low self-esteem, obsessive thoughts, winter blues, irritability and insomnia. Take 50 to 100 mg of the serotonin-boosting supplement 5-hydroxy-tryptophan (5-HTP) in consultation with your doctor.

FLAXSEED OIL - *reset your body's thermostat*

Alpha-linolenic acid (LNA) and other fatty acids found in flaxseed oil help reset your body's thermostat to a normal level and you start burning excess calories and also reduce sugar cravings. One tablespoon a day with a meal is the recommended dosage.

GLA - *activate brown fat*

Gamma-linolenic acid (GLA) helps you lose weight by activating dormant brown fat that helps burn excess calories.

CLA - *inhibit the enzyme that stores fat*

The essential fatty acid – conjugated linolenic acid (CLA) helps weight loss. It is seen, people who take 3000 milligrams of CLA daily lose about 20% of their body fat within three months without dieting.

FISH OIL - *helps balance overall fat intake*

A medical study reveals, fatty acids available in fish oil are unable to reduce weight directly but help in balancing your overall intake of fats and maintain good health. Consult a dietician for treatment.

Don't skip meals to burn fat

Fasting cleanses the body of all the imbedded waste matter, removes the deep-rooted toxins and gives rest to the different organs of the body. To begin fasting, eat only raw vegetables or fruits. Do not take more than four to five glasses of liquid diet a day. Take only fresh lime with honey or plain water. Never begin or end fasting suddenly. For the next four to five days take only raw or boiled vegetables. Over a period of ten days you can come back to your original cereal diet. Apart from dieting, many of the ailments such as acne and pimples, rheumatism, asthma, ulcers, alcoholism, heart disease and many more disorders are cured.

Healthy eating pyramid

Follow 'healthy eating pyramid' guidelines, which recommends that between 35 and 40% of your diet should come from whole grains like cereals and brown bread, rice and pasta. Vegetables should form 15 to 25% of your daily intake, followed by fruits about 10 to 15%, then dairy products and meats, which should be only about 10% each. Added fats, oils and sweets should be no more than 5%.

The optimum diet plan

Follow these points carefully:

○ Overeating is a cumulative process and weight gain is the result. What you eat in a day or even a week won't make much difference, but over a year you will misjudge your food intake.

○ A balanced food makes you thinner. If your diet lacks adequate vitamins and minerals, your body will want to eat more to make up for the deficiency.

○ Slow weight loss is best. Reduce your daily calorie level only a little, no more than 20%. It means to lose around ½ kg to 1 kg a week. The problem with low-fat diets is that people are tempted to eat unlimited low-fat diets.

47

Essential supplements to fat burning

○ Eat healthy diet.

○ Regular exercise.

○ Amino acids and enzymes crucial to fat-metabolism may help you burn fat more efficiently.

○ Co-enzyme Q-10, a powerful nutrient is linked to every cell in the body. Q-10 aids energy production and possesses fat-burning properties.

○ Chromium Picolinate (amino acid) regulates insulin – the hormone that balances blood sugar levels.

○ Hydroxy-Citric Acid (HCA) encourages the production of glycogen from carbohydrates, which accumulates in the liver and muscles. It reduces appetite, increases energy levels in the body and helps the body burn existing fat to produce energy.

○ *Green Tea:* The body has two types of fat: Brown and Yellow. Yellow fat is visible below the surface of the skin whereas Brown fat accumulates around the skeleton in the upper part of body and triggers the metabolism of stored yellow fat. The yellow fat increases calorie intake. Green tea helps melting fats.

○ *L-Carnitine:* An amino acid manufactured in the liver, has a vital role in helping the body transform fat into fuel. L-Carnitines greatly enhance properties when taken before exercise. 500 to 1000 mg. per day is the recommended dosage, which should be taken after consultation with your doctor.

○ *Lipotropic Factors:* Nutrients which function in the liver as fat prevent excessive build up of fat. Lipotropic factors are an aid to weight loss and help to reduce body fat and localised fat like cellulite.

○ *Omega-3:* These essential fatty acids reverse the weight gain, high cholesterol levels and risk of heart disease caused by saturated fats. Food rich in Omega-3 include fish oils, soyabeans, linseeds and walnuts, which help to reduce cholesterol and triglyceride levels, improve fat metabolism and aid weight loss. Vegetarians can take linseed oil instead of fish oil. (400 to 800 mg per day is the recommended dosage as per doctor's advice).

O *Sweating:* The fast way to burn fat.

Workout programmes for slimming: Muscle is a fat-burning furnace taking centimetres off your waistline. Low-intensity exercise is just as effective, but you will need to work out for longer in order to get results. Choose a fat-burning workout of your choice from different fat-burning regimes. Strenuous swimming burns four times more calories than strenuous running. 20 minutes on the stair climber followed by 20 minutes of sit-ups develops a high-intensity regime that tones and slims chest, shoulders, back, arms, legs and feet. A gym or health club is the perfect environment for exercising without distractions. Use the exercise bike, treadmill and rowing machine. A recent study showed that on every two kg. muscle you build, you burn an extra 30 to 50 calories a day. Skating provides a better aerobic workout than cycling. You burn an average 285 calories during a 30-minute period of skating. A good exercise programme will take into account not only the demands of your lifestyle but also of your body.

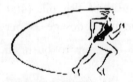

Chapter-6

Recommended Dietary Allowance Programme and Slimming

Anatomy and Physiology

To achieve good grooming, it is essential to have thorough knowledge of the working of human body and major body systems. The major body systems include integumentary system, skeletal system, muscular system, respiratory system, circulatory system, digestive system, genito-urinary system, nervous system and endocrine system.

The Cells: The human organism is made up of a vast variety of parts that vary in complexity, which include organ systems, organs, tissues and cells. The cell is the basic structure from which all other body structures are made. These are the basic units of all living things, including bacteria, plants and animals. The human body is composed entirely of cells made up of protoplasm – a colourless, jelly-like substance in which food elements such as protein, fats, carbohydrates, mineral salts and water are present. As long as the cell receives an adequate supply of food, oxygen and water; eliminates waste products and is favoured with proper temperature; it will continue to grow and thrive. However, in case these conditions do not exist and there is the presence of toxins (poison), the cells are impaired.

Metabolism is a chemical process in which the cells are nourished and supplied with energy to carry on many activities in the human body. In a healthy body, the metabolic rate is kept under control by a secretion from the thyroid gland. Body tissues are composed of group of cells. Each tissue has a specific function and can be recognised by its characteristic appearance. They are of various types: Connective tissue (Fat tissues) to support, protect and bind together body tissues; Muscular tissue contracts and moves various parts of the body; Nerve tissue controls and coordinates all body functions; Epithelial tissue such as skin, mucous, membranes, linings of heart, digestive and respiratory organs and glands; and Liquid tissue carry food, waste products and hormones by means of the blood and lymph.

Organs are structures designed to accomplish a definite function. The important organs of the body are the brain, heart, lungs, liver, kidneys, the stomach and intestines.The skeleton of human body is divided into three main regions: the skull, the spine and the limbs. The blood carries oxygen from the respiratory system and nutrients from the digestive system to the cells.

Metabolism is a series of chemical reactions, which utilises the nutrients for growth, repair or energy production within the body. Metabolism is the rate at which the body uses energy. Energy is measured in kilocalories (kcal) or kilojoules. One calorie is the amount of energy required to raise the temperature of 1 kg of water by 1 degree C. Joule is the metric unit of measurement for heat and energy (1 kcal : 4.2 kj) The energy value of nutrients such as carbohydrates is 3.75 kcal (16 kj), protein is 4.00 kcal (17 kj) and fat is 9.00 kcal (37 kj)

What is the requirement of energy in human body

The amount of food which a person requires depends on the energy used each day. This varies according to age, sex, body structure, occupation, physical activities and conditions such as pregnancy or health. In fact, the food eaten in a day should not supply more or less than the required amount of energy used in the day. The average energy requirements for an average adult woman should be approximately 1940 kcal, and for an adult man 2550 kcal.

51

Various occupations and activities

Sedentary	Office workers, teachers and shop workers.
Moderate activities	Hairdressers, beauticians and postmen.
Very active jobs	Construction labourers, athletes and hockey/football players.
Leisure activities	Jogging.
Special needs	Extra energy is required during the final months of pregnancy and breastfeeding.

Basal metabolic rate (BMR)

This is the amount of energy required to keep the body alive when it is warm and at complete rest. Women, elderly people, females during periods and menopause tend to have a lower BMR than men because they have less muscle tissue. The BMR is also lower in elderly people and during periods of starvation, when the body needs lower food energy. The average value of BMR for a woman aged 40 is 1360 kcal (5700 kj), and a man of age 40 is 1750 kcal (7300 kj) per day.

As an example, the table below illustrates the energy used for various activities (25-year-old in sitting job weighing 62 kg).

Activity	Kcal/hour	kj used/hour
Sleeping	57	238
Sitting (eating)	66	300
Standing (cooking)	126	540
Washing and dressing	126	540
Walking moderately quickly	210	900
Walking up/down stairs	390	1620
Office sitting	90	360
Office walking	156	660
Dancing	270	1140
Average jogging	390	1620

When to seek advice of a doctor

○ If the age is under 18 or over 70 years.

○ When undergoing medical treatment.

○ In case of severe obesity.

○ On a medically prescribed diet.

○ In case of pregnancy or feeding a child.

Diet advice for weight loss

1. The best way to lose weight is to combine a diet with an exercise programme.

2. Aim for a small, steady weight loss of half or one kg per week.

3. Avoid crash diets.

4. Other than a reduction in energy content, the diet must be well balanced.

5. Eat at least three meals a day, so that energy intake is spread evenly.

6. Try to avoid eating in between meals.

7. Drink plenty of fluids.

8. Include treats, occasionally, as reward.

Recommended dietary allowance for expecting mothers

The recommended dietary allowance (RDA) suggests the following major nutrients. A adult woman should consume approximately 1900 to 2200 kcal/day and a man approximately 2200 to 2500 kcal/day as daily energy requirement. However, during pregnancy and breastfeeding, energy requirements are higher and a woman needs between 2200 to 2500 kcal/day. These requirements should be supplemented by a balanced combination of carbohydrates, protein, vegetables, and fat in moderation. The keyword here is quality and not quantity.

53

It's not how much you eat but what you eat. The following nutrients are required during pregnancy or lactation period:

Nutrient	Daily requirement	Development	Rich source
Protein	65 gm	overall growth	pulses, dairy products and soya bean.
Calcium	1000 mg	bones and teeth	dairy products, soya bean products, green leafy vegetables.
Iron	40 mg	red blood cells	dried beans, cereals and pulses and dry fruits.
Folic acid	400 mcg	early stage of pregnancy and breastfeeding	potatoes, cereals, nuts, pulses and soya bean.
Fat	30 gm	enhance energy	
Vitamin C	40 mg	bones, cartilage, muscles and blood vessels	citrus fruits, amla and vegetables
Vitamin A	2400 mcg	healthy skin	yellow/orange, vegetables (carrot and pumpkin), fruit (mango, papaya) and whole milk.
Vitamin D	through sunlight	aids the absorption of calcium in body	sunlight, certain fish
Vitamin B12	non-veg. food		soya milk and products
Iodine	iodised salt	baby's brain in foetus	cereals (rice, wheat, jowar) nuts and oilseeds (til, etc.)

Do's and don'ts

O Use fresh fruits and vegetables which are most nutritious.

O Refrigerated foods for long period result in loss of vital nutrients.

O Eat unpeeled fruits and vegetables (like potatoes, cucumber and carrot) so that the body receives right amount of fibre and nutrients.

O Do not soak vegetables in water for longer periods of time to avoid loss of water-soluble vitamins B and C.

O Cook vegetables carefully so that they retain most of their nutrients during cooking process.

O Prepare fresh salad or raita just before taking meal.

O Include a large amount of sprouts in your diet, which aids in easy digestion.

O Avoid using soda bi-carbonate while cooking as it destroys essential nutrients.

Diet recommended during breastfeeding

During breastfeeding you will require a lot more calories than you did during your pregnancy. Breastfeeding will make you burn 3500 kcal per day. However, you need to consume only 2400 to 2700 kcal during the first six months of lactation if you are exclusively breastfeeding your baby. Your energy requirement will decrease to 2250 to 2550 kcal per day after six months of lactation period when you will begin to wean your baby. The following nutrients are required during lactation:

O *Protein:* during first six months of lactation the requirement will be 75 gm/day, and after six months the requirement will reduce to 68 gm/day.

O *Fat:* daily requirement is 45 gm.

O *Calcium:* 1000 mg/day. Breast milk is a great source of calcium for development of bones in mother as well as child.

○ *Iron:* 30 mg/day, that supplies oxygen to each cell of the human body.

○ *Folic acid:* 150 mcg/day, which is essential for the growth and development of the brain and spine of the baby.

○ *Vitamin C:* 80 mg/day, required for the formation of collagen and also for immunity against infections and diseases.

○ *Vitamin A (Beta-carotene):* 3800 mcg/day.

○ *Vitamin D:* necessary to absorb calcium in the body.

Healthy diets

Quick garlic soup – 6 calories per serving

Ingredients for 5 cups:

❖ 5 cups water

❖ 4-6 garlic cloves (minced)

❖ ½ teaspoon each ground sage and dried thyme

❖ 2 tablespoons fresh parsley (chopped)

❖ 1 bay leaf and salt to taste

Bring water to a boil. Add garlic, sage, thyme, salt, bay leaf and parsley. Simmer for 15 minutes. Adjust seasoning. Can be reheated while taking.

Quick vegetable soup – 65 calories per serving

Ingredients for 2 cups:

❖ 1½ cups water

❖ ¼ cup green beans (chopped)

❖ ½ cup each cabbage (shredded), turnips, zucchini, yellow squash and fresh parsley (chopped)

❖ 1 medium size tomato (chopped)

❖ ½ teaspoon each dried thyme, rosemary and marjoram

❖ Seasoning vegetable and salt to taste

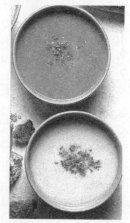

Bring water to a boil in a saucepan. Add the parsnips and green beans. Simmer for 4-5 minutes. Add cabbage, zucchini and squash. Simmer for a few minutes more. Add the parsley, tomato, thyme, rosemary, marjoram, seasoning vegetable and salt. Simmer a few minutes. Remove from heat and adjust seasoning.

Gazpacho – 115 calories per serving
Mix together all ingredients for 4 servings:
- ❖ 4 ripe tomatoes, peeled and diced
- ❖ 1 small onion, very finely diced
- ❖ 1 cucumber, peeled and finely diced
- ❖ 1 green bell pepper, very finely diced
- ❖ 1 red bell pepper, very finely diced
- ❖ ½ carrot, very finely diced
- ❖ 2 garlic cloves, minced
- ❖ 10 fresh basil leaves
- ❖ 2 tablespoons parsley, finely chopped
- ❖ 1 tablespoon olive oil
- ❖ ¼-½ cup fresh lemon juice
- ❖ 2 cups cold tomato juice
- ❖ salt and pepper to taste and red pepper sauce (opt.)

Cucumber, tomato and yogurt salad – 110 calories
Ingredients for 4 servings:
- ❖ 3 cups nonfat plain yogurt
- ❖ 2 small ripe tomatoes (seeded and chopped)
- ❖ 1 small cucumber (peeled, seeded, shredded)
- ❖ 1 small onion (minced)
- ❖ 1 fresh green chili pepper (seeded and sliced)
- ❖ 3 tablespoons fresh coriander (chopped)
- ❖ salt to taste

Place the yogurt in a bowl and whisk with a fork until creamy and smooth. Add tomatoes, cucumber, onion, chili pepper, coriander and salt.

Garden pasta salad – 225 calories

Ingredients for 8 servings:

- ❖ 450 gm corkscrew pasta
- ❖ ½ cup red onion (diced)
- ❖ 1 zucchini squash (finely diced)
- ❖ 6 radishes (trimmed and diced)
- ❖ 2 large ripe tomatoes (cored, seeded and diced)
- ❖ 1 green bell pepper (finely diced)
- ❖ 1 red bell pepper (finely diced)
- ❖ ¼ cup fresh parsley (finely chopped)

Cook pasta only. Run under cold water. Mix all vegetables in a large bowl. Toss salad with dressing of choice.

Basil lime chicken salad – 175 calories

Ingredients for 4 servings:

- ❖ 4 cups chicken stock
- ❖ ½ cup chopped fresh basil
- ❖ ¼ cup fresh lime juice
- ❖ 4 skinless, boneless chicken breasts (cut in half)
- ❖ freshly ground pepper, to taste
- ❖ pinch of salt

Combine the chicken stock, basil, lime juice, pepper and salt. Pour into a frying pan in one layer. Bring liquid to boil. Layer chicken in liquid without overlapping. Cover and simmer for about 4 minutes. Remove from heat and allow to cool at room temperature. Refrigerate overnight. Slice and toss in a green salad with vinaigrette.

Pasta – 335 calories

Ingredients for 6 servings:

- ❖ 10 sun-dried tomatoes
- ❖ 400 gm spinach fettuccine
- ❖ 2 tablespoons olive oil
- ❖ 2 garlic cloves (minced or crushed)

- ❖ 1 medium onion (chopped)
- ❖ ½ cup each red bell pepper and mushrooms (sliced)
- ❖ 1 cup spinach (coarsely chopped)
- ❖ ½ teaspoon ground nutmeg
- ❖ salt and pepper to taste

Put sun-dried tomatoes in a bowl. Pour boiling water over them to cover. Let stand for about 15 minutes or until tomatoes are tender. Drain tomatoes and discard liquid. Cut tomatoes into strips. Cook the pasta and drain. Heat the olive oil in a saucepan. Add to it garlic, onion and red bell pepper. Leave for about 3 minutes. Add mushroom and spinach. Stir for one minute. Now mix to it sun-dried tomatoes, pasta, nutmeg, salt and pepper. Cook and stir for about two minutes or until heated through. Toss vegetables over pasta.

Precautions:

- ○ Do not overcook, in order to save calories.
- ○ All pasta should be firm, not soft and mushy.

Lemon rice – 310 calories

Ingredients for 8 servings:
- ❖ 2 tablespoons olive oil
- ❖ 1 onion (finely chopped)
- ❖ 3 cups white rice
- ❖ 2 cups chicken stock
- ❖ 1 cup water
- ❖ juice of 3 lemons
- ❖ 5 lemon slices
- ❖ 1 teaspoon sea salt
- ❖ 2 bay leaves
- ❖ 4 whole cloves
- ❖ freshly ground pepper to taste

Heat the olive oil in a medium saucepan. Add to it onion. Stir in the rice coating the grains with the oil. Stir for 4-5 minutes.

Meanwhile, in a saucepan combine the chicken stock, water, lemon juice, lemon slices, salt, pepper, bay leaves and cloves. Bring to a boil. Stir this mixture into the rice. Cover and simmer over low heat for 15 to 20 minutes.

Mashed sweet potatoes – 275 calories

Ingredients for 4 servings:

- ❖ 5 large sweet potatoes (scrubbed)
- ❖ 1 cup low-fat milk
- ❖ 2 teaspoons butter
- ❖ ¼ teaspoon each nutmeg and cinnamon
- ❖ 1 teaspoon salt
- ❖ freshly ground black pepper to taste
- ❖ 1 to 2 teaspoons balsamic vinegar

Preheat oven to 400° F. Bake the sweet potatoes for about 50 minutes, until easily pierced with a fork. Peel and mash potatoes by hand. Now heat the butter in a saucepan over low flame until it browns. Stir in the nutmeg and cinnamon. Remove from the heat and stir in the milk. Add the sweet potato puree and mix thoroughly. Pour over salt and pepper. Stir in balsamic vinegar.

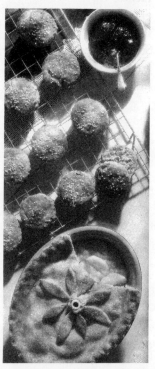

Chicken with garlic sauce – 340 calories

Ingredients for 4 servings:

- ❖ 1 tablespoon olive oil
- ❖ ½ cup dry white wine
- ❖ 4 boneless, skinless chicken breast halves
- ❖ 4 garlic cloves (minced or pressed)
- ❖ ¼ cup fresh Italian parsley (chopped)

Heat the olive oil in a large nonstick frying pan. Add to it garlic. After a minute mix in it chicken and continue stirring. Add wine and bring to a boil. Lower heat, cover the pan and cook for about 5 minutes. Garnish with fresh parsley.

Apple-rice pudding – 120 calories

Ingredients for 8 servings:

- ❖ 1½ cups low-fat milk
- ❖ 2 cups cooked rice (brown or white) and peeled apple
- ❖ 3 egg whites
- ❖ 2 tablespoons sugar
- ❖ 2 teaspoons vanilla
- ❖ ½ teaspoon each orange peel (grated) and cinnamon
- ❖ 1/3 cup dried apricots (chopped)
- ❖ 1/8 teaspoon nutmeg

Preheat oven to 325° F. Combine milk, egg whites, sugar, vanilla, orange peel and cinnamon. Beat with an electric mixer until smooth. Stir in rice, apples and apricot. Sprinkle with nutmeg. Spoon into 8 custard cups, then place cups in pan filled with hot water. Bake until browned for 50-60 minutes. Remove cups from the water and allow to cool.

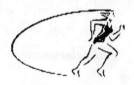

Chapter-7

Massage Programme for Slimming

Massage treatment for weight loss

Massage treatment is very useful to melt extra fat from the body, especially in women after the age of 50, during pregnancy, and after childbirth. Practice the following steps:

○ Squeeze either side of the wrist above the wrist bone.

○ Press on the hollow inside the ankles just behind the bony prominence.

○ Press in the middle of the groove between nose and upper lip.

To fight overweight, pay attention on the fleshiest areas of the body such as abdomen, thighs and buttocks using stimulating movements such as kneading and pummeling. Vigorous massage helps in slimming. Remember, massage alone without regular exercise and control over the diet cannot reduce weight or break down fat. Massage tones the skin, soothes the body, produces energy by stimulating the circulation. Weight watchers should concentrate on self-body massage of the following fleshiest areas:

○ *Abdomen:* Lie on your back and knead abdomen thoroughly.

○ *Hips:* Roll on to one side; knead and pummel both hips.

○ *Thighs:* Sit up and knead thighs from knees up to the hips vigorously.

○ *Buttocks:* Pummel fast over thighs up to the buttocks.

Massage for brides before marriage

In case of a heavy figure with fat deposits over abdomen, hips, thighs and buttocks, a proper daily massage is essential at the time of bath two to three weeks before marriage. Massage with a massaging cream has miraculous effect on the skin. A special recipe (paste) for brides to be used daily can be prepared by mixing the following ingredients and rubbing it thoroughly to stimulate the skin:

Dried ground lemon peel	1 tablespoon
Almond powder	½ tablespoon
Wheat-germ flour	4 tablespoons
Ground thyme	1 tablespoon
Almond oil	3-4 drops
Jasmine oil	3-4 drops
Salt	a pinch

Rub on the body thoroughly for 30 minutes before taking bath.

Massage for expectant mothers

Careful, smooth and gentle massage movements benefit during the period of pregnancy. Massage helps alleviate many complications such as tension, backache, insomnia and fatty deposits on the body. Avoid deep pressure and percussion. A careful massage is definitely beneficial during pregnancy and before conception to increase the fertility of a woman. Use all stroking techniques for massaging abdomen, back, shoulders, legs and foot massage ensuring very light and gentle strokes. Massage done by a trained masseuse makes childbirth easier. Lower back and shoulders are the areas to concentrate for relieving tension while massaging. The

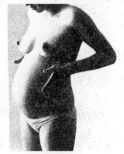
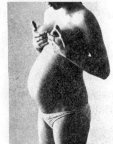

various massage movements for a pregnant woman include gentle strokes on the abdomen with hands, one following the other clockwise. Stroke softly on the sides of the stomach based upwards with hands, one following the other till hands reach the navel. Then glide hands gently towards abdomen. Cup your hands over the navel for few seconds until you feel the heat, then lift hands slowly. A regular abdomen massage makes child delivery easy and painless.

Leg massage during pregnancy: is especially beneficial, soothing, relaxing, relieving swelling and pain in legs. Varicose veins or cramps in the leg muscles are common problems often faced by expectant women. Such women should always sleep with legs and feet slightly raised above the level of head. This sleeping posture relieves swollen legs by aiding manual lymph drainage. The lymphatic pumping system drains off the waste products from the body and ensures circulation of purified blood in the body. Besides slimming and eliminating wastes from the body, backache, morning sickness, the massage helps in strengthening the immune system curing many skin disorders like acne, eczema, dermatitis and skin inflammation.

Arms and back massage during pregnancy: Arms massage during this period leaves soothing effect on the body when restrictions of abdomen massage are advised for expectant mothers. Backache and morning sickness are the common complaints during pregnancy, which can be relieved to a great extent with back massage. Avoid deep pressure to the lower back. Back pain can be alleviated with plenty of smooth and flowing stroking movements on the mid back, just above the waist, at the base of spine, and between shoulder blades. Press firmly by applying circular pressure with your thumb on the hips and buttocks.

Massage after childbirth

Massage of abdomen for 40 days after the delivery of baby energises the mother, cures body aches, sheds extra flesh and brings uterus to the original position prior to delivery.

To give an abdomen massage to women after childbirth, the following steps should be applied:

○ Stroke the abdomen in all directions.

○ Knead firmly on hips, gently across the abdomen.

○ Stroke clockwise in large circles on the abdomen applying gentle pressure.

○ Stroke slowly up on the lower abdomen starting from the pubic bone to the navel.

○ Cup hands over the navel for a few seconds until you feel heat under the hands. Then lift hands slowly.

When massaging the face

○ Wash hands with soap before starting massage.

○ Remove all traces of stale or fresh make-up before massage otherwise the skin pores will get blocked.

○ Remove blackheads before massage.

○ Remove oiliness with cleansing milk or pH acid, if the skin is too oily. Use moisturiser before massage, if the skin is over dry. Use astringent lotion before massage, if the skin is damp and fleshy.

○ The best time to massage the face is at night before going to sleep.

○ Start massage from the neck upward and end at the forehead or temples because all veins and tissues get blood circulation.

○ Avoid pressing the delicate skin around the eyes.

○ Massage for a minimum of 15-20 minutes as cream takes that much time to get absorbed.

○ Always wipe off extra cream with a cotton swab.

How to massage the face

Blend a little cleansing cream with the fingers to soften it. Using both hands apply cream over the face following these massage movements:

- ○ Start at the chin and with a sweeping movement slide to end of jaw.
- ○ Continue from base of nose to temple, along the side of nose, between the brows, and across forehead to temples.
- ○ Now take additional cream, blend it, smooth down the neck, chest and back.
- ○ Next, start massaging at the centre of forehead, move lightly around eyes, then towards temples and back to the centre of the forehead.
- ○ Slide down from nose to upper lip, smooth to temples and forehead, then move lightly down to chin and finally slide up towards jaw line, temples and forehead.
- ○ Remove cream with cleansing tissues or warm, moist towel.
- ○ Emollient cream selected according to skin type should be applied in the same manner as indicated above.
- ○ Use lanolin or hormone cream for a dry skin and cold cream for an oily skin.
- ○ For neck, face, shoulder and chest, apply emollient cream.

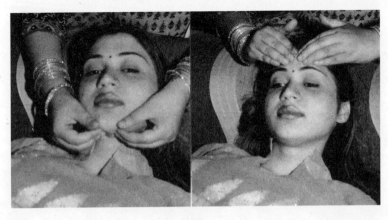

- Apply eye cream under the eyes gently with fingertips.
- Use muscle oil around the neck.
- For massaging face, apply a massage cream giving manipulations using slightly cupped hands and fingers. Start massage under the lower lip with two fingers. Repeat process several times. Pinch gently along the jaw line, working towards the ears.

Why massage

Massage is one of the easiest ways for attaining and maintaining health, youth, vigour, beauty, melting extra fat and relieving tension and stress. According to an expert's advice, when couples touch each other and embrace, it can prevent physical and mental illness. It improves circulation, relaxes muscles, aids digestion by stimulating the lymphatic system, eliminates waste products, provides energy, refreshes and revitalises body. The word 'massage' has been derived from the Arabic word 'Masah' – which means 'the magic of hands.'

Important tips for massage

- Early morning massage has a miraculous effect on the various organs. To get beneficial results, it is important that massage is given in a comfortable environment. Choose a warm, peaceful place with dim lights.
- Always lie on a firm, padded surface to relax the back and the stomach. Place a cushion under the knees to reduce the arch of the lower back and place a small cushion or folded towel under the head.
- A hard bed is ideal if you want to give a soothing massage, which can leave you relaxed and sleepy.
- Keep your back straight throughout the massage and use the weight of your body to give rhythm and depth.
- Never stay in one position when massaging.
- Wear loose-fitting washable clothes and be bare-footed.

- Remove ornaments before massage; they can cause scratches.
- Support a sway back with a cushion under the waist.
- If you feel pain or an uncomfortable situation during massage, inform the masseur.
- Mould your hands to the contours of the body.
- Vary pressure from very light to very strong. The massage should be lighter over bony areas and firmer over the muscles. Do not apply heavy pressure when massaging.
- Concentrate on the massage. Avoid talking when massaging. Feel totally relaxed for a good massage.
- Do not worry if your initial movements seem clumsy. Practice will make you perfect.

Avoid massage, if you suffer from

- An infection or a contagious skin disease.
- High temperature.
- Skin infection, bruises or an acute inflammation.
- An inflammatory condition such as thrombosis or phlebitis.
- Inflammatory cases of joints.
- Infectious diseases like diphtheria and gonorrhoea which cause formation of pus; a massage may spread the pus to the entire system.
- During pregnancy without consulting your doctor.

Few massage techniques

- *Reflexology massage* (75-minute treatment): Finger pressure is applied to the reflex points of feet to stimulate the related organs of the body and to restore balance in muscular systems.

○ *Relaxing massage* (50-minute treatment): It relieves stress, reduces muscle fatigue and improves blood circulation resulting in shedding extra fat deposits.

○ *Therapeutic massage:* An ideal massage for toning the muscles, treatment of sensitive areas affected by muscular tension, stress and fatigue.

○ *Sports massage* (50-minute treatment): It helps to reduce muscle fatigue and eliminates toxins produced in the muscles during physical exercise.

○ *Anti-cellulite massage:* A reductive massage that works in parts with the highest concentration of cellulite. It generates heat to help dissolve body fat. Excellent results are obtained when it is followed by a sauna session (steam bath) and completed with a shower bath.

○ *Lymphatic drainage:* A massage technique, which helps to detoxify the skin of the body. This massage movement helps to drain toxins, prevent fatness and control premature ageing.

○ *Shiatsu-massage:* A massage technique in which 'Shi' means finger and 'Atsu' means the pressure. In this movement, the fingers, palms and sometimes elbows are used to exercise pressure on a few pressure points of the body to stimulate energy. This massage technique reduces stress, alleviates aches, pains, fatigue and fat deposits on the body.

○ *Ultrasonic massage therapy:* It helps to provide glow, improve dry dull and sallow skins, improve blood circulation and activate sebaceous glands. It is a highly effective massage treatment to slim the body; especially beneficial in winter season.

○ *Suction massage therapy:* It sucks out infection, harmful bacteria, dirt, dust, germs from the upper layer of the epidermis and from the deeper stratum. The benefits of this massage include tightening of the skin, leaving it germs-free, helping to control sebum, improves blood circulation and removes infection.

○ *Thai massage:* A massage therapy recognised as an effective means of reducing stress, pain, promotes muscular and general relaxation, recovery from injury, circulation of blood and lymph and restoration of metabolic balance. Thai massage is a combination of acupressure, breathing technique, gentle stretches and beautiful postures.

Rejunvenation therapies

Siddha Vaidya and Ayurveda are useful therapies in which special herbal oils are used to achieve balance in the overall body. They affect the autonomic nervous system, the endocrine system, blood pressure, make body slim and trim, relieve stress, increase protein biosynthesis, elevate body enzyme synthesis, improve mental power, increase physical ability, fight free radicals, improve eyesight, are beneficial to cardio-vascular and respiratory system.

Shirodhara, nasya, rasayanas, abhyanga (massage), svedana (steaming), sneha (application of pastes and masks), aromatherapy (massage with herbal oils), chromotherapy (treatment with colour therapy), panchkarma (scientific system to detoxify and rejuvenate whole body), kriya karma (rejuvenation), purva karma, crystal and gem therapy, ozone therapy (treatment by producing alkaline rays), micro therapy, (power massage to improve blood circulation, stimulate nerves and muscles and regenerate cells and tissues), high frequency therapy (thermal heat produced due to rapid vibrations but without muscular contraction), derma-brasion (to remove uneven tone), shirobasti, akashi tarpan (treatment with medicated ghee or oil in eyes), juice therapy, siddha massage are some of naturopathic therapies beneficial for the body.

What is lymphatic massage

This massage technique helps in purifying the blood from the heart (on left side) and lymphatic ducts that exist on right side through 18 lymphatic nodes in human body. Lymphatic massage has a number of advantages.

70

- The waste products are released from the body.
- Helps fight bacteria and infections, and removes waste matter from tissues.
- Improves blood circulation.
- Melts extra fat deposits in the body.
- Relaxes nodes.
- The waste fluids get removed from the veins through urine.
- Excellent for curing acne and skin diseases.

Following precautions are essential during lymphatic massage:

- Lie straight for lymphatic massage.
- Avoid massage if the age is below 16 years.
- Wrongly done massage is harmful; may cause vomiting and headache.
- Massage can be done on every type of skin.
- Remove make-up before massage and cleanse the skin thoroughly.
- The massage movements should be carried by touch therapy (effleurage movement) or with the help of electrical gadgets.

Body massage

Massage is a scientific method of giving manipulations to the body by rubbing, pinching, kneading, tapping or stroking with the hands and fingers using various types of massage creams and oils available in the market. Body massage has the following benefits:

- Stimulates and smoothens the nerves.
- Relieves body tension.
- Increases circulation of blood.

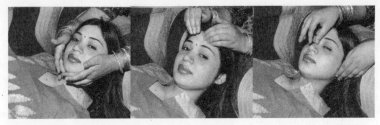

○ Causes muscle contraction.

○ Stimulates the action of skin glands.

○ Helps to relieve pain in the muscles.

○ Softens the skin.

○ Calms, relaxes and relieves emotional tension.

○ And above all, it alleviates and melts fat.

Precautions when massaging

○ Do not massage over an area where redness, swelling, pus is present.

○ Don't break contact with skin until massage is finished.

○ Always massage towards origin of the muscles.

○ Keep fingernails short to avoid scratching the skin.

○ Carry out massage rhythmically from the insertion to the origin of muscles.

○ Massaging in wrong direction causes muscles and skin to sag.

Some don'ts

Massage should not be done in following conditions:

○ Heart diseases.

○ High blood pressure.

○ Inflamed or swollen joints.

○ Glandular swelling.

○ Abrasions of the skin.

○ A skin disease.

○ Broken capillaries.

Some do's while massaging

○ A firm, sure touch.

○ Develop strong, flexible hands.

○ Self control.

○ Quiet temperament.

○ Use of psychology.

○ Trimmed nails and warm, dry hands.

Massage movements to slim body

Effleurage (Stroking movement): This is light, stroking, continuous movement applied with the palms and fingers in slow and rhythmic manner (without applying pressure). This massage movement is applied to melt fat on the forehead, face, neck, chest, shoulders, back, arms and hands. While massaging, the hand is held loosely, the wrist is kept flexible and fingers should conform to the shape of the area being massaged.

Petrissage (Kneading movement): This movement involves palm of hands, pads of fingers and thumbs, and applied with light but firm pressure. This massage movement promotes blood circulation and helps in melting fat on back, shoulder and thighs. This massage technique softens and relaxes hard contracted muscles, eliminates fatigue, stimulates sensory nerves, increases blood and lymph circulation and helps to tone and strengthen muscles.

Tapotement (or Percussion): In this massage technique comprising of tapping, slapping and hacking movements, the pressure is applied with the sides of hand with partly flexed fingers or fingertips. This massage movement effects increase in blood circulation, strengthens and tone the muscles, stimulates sensory nerves, increases lymph circulation and redistributes fatty tissue.

Friction (Deep rubbing movement): Light circular movement produced by the pads or fingertips or thumbs of the hands, used on the scalp, arms, face and neck. This movement breaks down nodules and fibrous adhesion, increases blood and lymph circulation, and slims down arms and legs.

73

Vibration (Shaking) Movement: A fine trembling movement always given along a nerve path with rapid muscular contractions using pad of fingers and thumb. Massaging in the wrong direction can cause muscles and skin to sag. Vibration movement has beneficial effects: it stimulates the nerves, loosens scar tissues, stretches adhesion and relieves pain.

Shiatsu therapy

Also known as acupressure therapy, it is used to treat disorders by pressing each pressure point on the body for three to five seconds. There are nearly 600 Shiatsu Points on the human body, which produce energy that flows in the body. It takes about 45 to 60 minutes to treat the whole body. Prominent pressure points exist on either side of the spine, abdomen, centre of the chest, buttocks, back and front of the legs, arms and hands. The following precautions are to be observed:

○ Keep arms straight, exerting pressure from shoulders.

○ Apply pressure with the balls of thumb and fingers.

○ Increase pressure steadily and evenly.

○ Keep knees apart and swing hips forward to apply gradual pressure.

○ Apply pressure lightly, steadily and evenly on abdomen especially in case of pregnant women.

○ The lighting should be dimmed. Many people like to hear music while having massage, others enjoy it in total peace and quiet, and a few may like to talk. The best is gentle music that suits most tastes.

○ Remove all clothes before massage for better treatment.

Aroma massage

Essential oils have a therapeutic effect on the body as they are analgesic, antibiotic, anti-fungal, anti-inflammatory, antioxidant, antiseptic, anti-spasmodic, anti-viral, carminative, depurative, digestive, diuretic, expectorant, hepatic, laxative, hypersensitive, sedative, stimulant and toning. Essential oils help to restore balance to the emotions and mind, which are capable to:

○ Soothe nervous tension and worries.

○ Melt extra fat.

○ Improve concentration and memory.

○ Uplift depression and negativity.

○ Induce deep relaxation, relieving both physical and mental fatigue.

○ Improve circulation to the muscles, thereby inducing inflammation and pain.

○ Release neck and shoulder tension and backache.

○ Relieve neuralgic arthritis and rheumatic conditions.

○ Help sprains, fractures, breaks, and heals easily.

○ Promote correct posture and help improve mobility.

○ Improve the function of every internal organ.

○ Improve digestion, assimilation and elimination.

○ Relieve constipation.

○ Increase the ability of the kidneys to function efficiently.

○ Flush the lymphatic system by the mechanical elimination of toxins and waste matter.

○ Reduce high blood pressure.

○ Help disperse headaches or migraines.

○ Stimulate mind and body without any side effect.

○ Stimulate the immune system.

○ Help relieve suppressed feelings.

○ Encourage deep breathing.

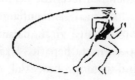

Chapter-8

Weight Loss Exercise Programme

An active lifestyle is the key to maintain your body, vitality and a youthful look. Those leading a sedentary lifestyle look older and lethargic resulting in premature ageing. If you want to stay young with attractive slim body, choose an exercising programme according to your age. There are people in their late 50s who look as good as if they were in their late 30s. Women who should be at the prime of youth in 30s sometimes look like they are in their 50s. We should no longer assume it as merely the luck of genetics or the result of a pampered lifestyle. Mind you, timely steps to maintain your body with suitable exercise programme can leave it flexible, slim and trim till the end. With body-friendly sculpt and tone workout you may chisel away the extra flab and optimise your physical and mental health.

What are warm up exercises

Perform low-impact aerobic moves for 5-10 minutes after a warm up and before beginning the workout. The best pre-stretch warm up is a five minute, low-impact march on the spot. Take a quick walk around your residential place or dance to your favourite tunes. The aim is to raise your core body temperature. After the warm up, stretch the body muscles and move into the exercise routine. Low-impact aerobic exercise include brisk walking, swimming and cycling – all excellent and gentle on the joints, maintain flexibility and help you stay in shape. Include some form of strength training to maintain strong muscles for good skeletal support.

What is weight loss programme

Most weight loss programmes recommend exercise as a means to burn excess calories. Unfortunately, many of these programmes fail to bring desired result due to unbalanced plan disturbing the balance of serotonin and insulin. The right kind of programme assists any weight loss programme, not only does it relieve stress and help prevent depression, it also corrects imbalances in blood sugar and insulin. It also helps inhibit fat formation. However, never overdo exercise. Unfortunately, many dieting women attack their bodies with such a fury of exercise that prolactin, serotonin and other important hormones go into the stress mode. All you need is about 30 minutes of exercise per day. If you can do more, gradually build up to a higher level. A weight loss programme doesn't recommend high-intensity exercise. You should follow these guidelines when selecting a programme:

○ Find an exercise you enjoy.

○ Exercise for at least thirty minutes, five times a week.

○ Never exercise to exhaustion.

○ Repetitive muscle movements are most effective at elevating serotonin.

○ Aerobics, walking, running and dancing are very effective forms of exercise.

○ Ancient 'Hatha Yoga' and 'Tai Chi' are excellent forms of exercise based on a balanced approach to fitness used for the entire mind-body connection.

○ Meditation is the ultimate way to reduce stress, lower heart rate and blood pressure. It reduces the hormones associated with stress – prolactin and glucocorticoids. Meditation lowers the thyroid-stimulating hormones creating depression and at the same time increases serotonin activity.

Weight loss programme for women in 20s

When you are in 20s, your metabolic rate is high enough to ensure that a low-fat diet, high in complex carbohydrates coupled with exercise will result in a beautiful body. Hormone levels are ensuring that bones can absorb calcium and increase in density besides gaining muscle mass. Muscle strength is at its peak and the lungs are at their maximum aerobic capacity. Body fat starts to increase and cholesterol levels are creeping up. It is time to get some good, vigorous exercises. A regular weight-bearing exercise helps ward off osteoporosis resulting in paying heavy dividends in later years. Mind this, excessive exercising and dieting can lead to a drop in oestrogen, which means an irreversible loss of bone density and a higher risk of developing osteoporosis.

Best exercise for burning fat includes aerobic exercise such as cycling, jogging, speed walking, step workouts, hip-hop dancing and kick-boxing. Play some fast-paced outdoor games. This increases your fat-free mass or muscle, which burns more calories than fat during the exercise and afterwards when you will idle. An inactive woman starts to lose muscle mass because it slows down her metabolism and will store unused energy in the form of fat not only around hips, buttocks and thighs but around internal organs too. This will also increase the risk of heart disease later on. If you are a busy working woman or involved in family and have hardly 10 minutes to exercise everyday, seize the chance – it will pay handsome rewards in the long run.

Daily workout even for ten minutes will reap benefits. Link daily personal routines and domestic chores to certain exercises such as tightening leg lifts, stomach crunches while standing, pelvic floor contractions and contracting your buttocks while you drive. Bring some form of exercise into family time – be it a walk, a musical dancing game or a swim, exercising bike or a treadmill practice in a health club. If nothing else, walk for 10-15 minutes daily in the morning or evening and go for long walks on weekends. You don't need to walk fast. The longer you move the more fat you will burn. Along with 1200 mg of calcium a day, do weight bearing exercises like weight lifting, which works together to build bone density.

Weight loss programme for women in 30s

Overall muscle strength drops after the age of 30. Bone mass declines at the rate of one percent a year. The ratio of body fat to muscle increases, so watch out for extra flab. Cholesterol continues to rise, increasing your risk of heart disease. You may continue exercise programme as in case of age 20s. Pregnant women should switch to an exercise that doesn't stress the particular part of the body. Wrong eating habits lead to anaemia, hyperacidity and bowel problems. A sedentary lifestyle leads to the onset of obesity, joint problems, hypertension, diabetes, varicose veins and even heart disease.

Take proper diet care to nourish your body – to maintain the muscle and bone density and also to keep fat levels down. Make sure that your diet is high in complex carbohydrates. Don't skimp on protein, it keeps hunger at bay and is useful for muscle repair and maintenance. Calcium, too, plays an important part to help ward off osteoporosis. So opt for low-fat dairy products and leafy green vegetables or take supplements. Always do a pre-stretch warm up before exercise. Avoid strict dietary rules and follow these guidelines:

○ Eat until you are 80% satisfied.

○ Eat fresh food – preferably steamed, stir-fried or poached.

○ Avoid extremes of temperature.

○ If you are a non-vegetarian, eat lots of fish and small quantity of meat.

○ Avoid alcohol, which may lead to breast cancer.

○ Drink ample water – six to eight glasses a day.

○ Don't forget calcium intake. Nutritional experts prescribe a daily dose of 1200 mg.

○ Eat lots of garden vegetables, fruits, drink herbal tea.

○ Choose whole-wheat chapaties, bread, cereals and unpolished rice.

○ Opt for low-fat milk, yogurt and cheese.

- Fats, oil, sugar, desserts and pastries assume dangerous implications as you age.
- Sprinkle minimum quantity of salt in your food.
- Regular physical examination is a must, to monitor weight and detect chronic problems early. Get simple tests done for anaemia and diabetes.
- Avoid eating red meat, milk, eggs, fried foods and sweets.

Weight loss programme for women in 40s

Oestrogen levels begin to drop, making it easier for fat to accumulate around the stomach and waist. Height reduction starts in this age due to weakening of the skeletal structure. Cartilage can suffer wear and tear, so there is less cushioning for bones and joints. Your body is like a machine – if you leave it out carelessly, it will rust. Beat the signs of ageing. Breasts start to lose their firmness as we get older and often become heavy, wrinkled, concave and develop stretch marks. Breasts are made up mostly of fat, so any weight change will affect their shape. Exercising without a proper-fitted bra will result in stretch marks. Even a woman with small breasts will find her breasts grow rapidly in pregnancy. Breastfeeding is responsible for the 'concave' look many women have in their upper breasts. Nursing can leave them looking wrinkled and deflated. Wearing a properly fitted bra is the best anti-gravity device. A good bra supports the breasts and helps keep them in good shape. If there is any change in breast size during pregnancy, during periods or when lactating the child, make sure to have a correctly fitted bra.

Exercise can help build up supporting muscles in the area surrounding the breasts. Swimming is a good exercise for the breasts, but don't forget to wear a swimsuit or bikini with well-fitted cups. Avoid sleeping while wearing a bra. Surgery can make heavy breasts to look smaller. Breast augmentation involves an incision above the breast and putting a silicone or saline implant in this pocket. Mastopexy is a process in which excess skin of breasts is cut away. Ptosis correction is a process to get rid of slack skin to reduce sagging.

Weight loss programme for women after 50

Most of the physical changes we consider natural to ageing are actually due to environmental toxins, lack of exercise, poor diet, smoking, excessive drinking and hormonal fluctuations. The symptoms can be delayed or minimised with proper care.

Height reduction begins fast as your skeletal structure starts to weaken. The average woman shrinks about 50 mm by the time she reaches 70. Your lung capacity starts decreasing. By the time you reach 70, it decreases by 40%. The risk of disease rises as your white blood cells are less efficient in fighting off cancer cells and infections. As muscles, ligaments and tendons tighten, you tend to lose flexibility. Extra fat on bottom and thighs becomes a part of the ageing process.

Obesity is common at this age, especially among those who have neglected themselves in 30s and 40s. Menopause itself brings along various problems. It is the female hormone or oestrogen which is manufactured in the body for as long as the monthly cycle continues. Sexual dysfunction sets in the early 50s. There is also an increased chance of breast, cervical and uterine cancer in this age group. Oestrogen helps in maintaining strong bones. After 50, you will need to hike your intake of calcium through milk products, green vegetables and fruits. Soya is very useful at this age, for apart from proteins it also contains phyto-oestrogen, which acts like natural oestrogen in the body.

Women experience the greatest drop in bone mass, especially after menopause. Light aerobic exercises keep fat at bay, muscles intact. The growing age leaves ill effect over the body. The skin on the body and neck gets looser and less elastic. It becomes dry and itchy. Wrinkles become more obvious, brown spots and scaly patches may develop on the body's skin, pores become smaller, there is less sweat and oil production and the hair shafts become thinner and hair starts greying. An average woman puts on about 6-8 kg between her 40s and 70s. Wrong eating habits and lack of exercise usually shows up during this time.

81

Follow these guidelines:

○ Regular walk in the morning or evening.

○ There is misconception that yogic asanas are difficult to perform at this age. In fact, yoga is a good way to remain fit and healthy in the 50s and afterwards (if health permits). Seek consultation of a yoga teacher.

Some easy-to-do exercises for women over 50

1. *Chair Pose (Utkata Posture):* Stand straight. Keep feet and knees together. Bend knees as you lower your body down until your thighs are parallel to the floor and imagine you are sitting on a chair. Now stretch your arms upwards joining palms. Hold for 10 minutes. Repeat exercise 3-4 times. This exercise strengthens and slims the ankles, calves, arms, legs, ankles, inner thighs and back.

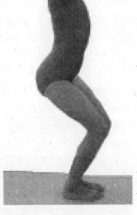

2. *Tara Posture:* This posture is divided into three positions:

   Position 1. Stand straight. Stretch your arms in front. Hold for 10-15 seconds.

   Position 2. Raise your arms straight over the head. Hold for 10-15 seconds.

   Position 3. Bring both arms on sides parallel to the ground. Hold for 10-15 seconds.

   This posture is especially useful for women above the age of 50 and pregnant women, being a light exercise. It has strengthening effect on lungs, chest and respiratory system.

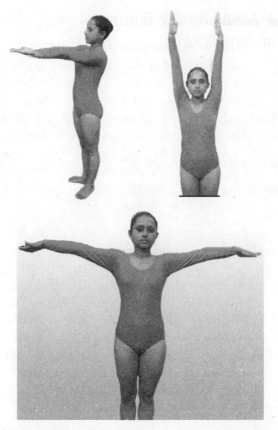

3. *Hasta Parshav Posture:* This exercise, too, is very useful for pregnant women. Lie on your back, arms on sides. Raise arms and rotate them clockwise in circles behind the head, inhaling. Repeat the exercise four times and gradually increase to ten times.

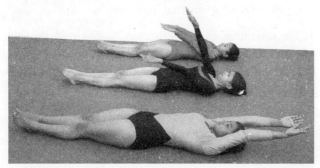

Exercise based on the mantra— 'no pain, much gain'

The exercise should be done with the mantra 'no pain, much gain'. Exercise is meant to be comfortable, healthy and happy – which should leave you fresh and ready to work, not wilting and ready for bed. From physical exercise one gets lightness, firmness, tolerance, elimination of impurities and stimulation of digestion. Exercising beyond a comfortable level leaves you feeling restless, exhausted and shaky. Avoid strain and pain exercises.

Exercise for 50% of your maximum capacity. If you can walk for one hour, go for 30 minutes. If you can run for 30 minutes, cut it down to 15 minutes so that your body doesn't have to repair it afterwards. If you have enough energy but tire quickly, go for very light exercises or walking. In winter, choose an indoor activity as extreme cold makes breathing difficult. Remember, you need exercising at comfortable level. If you are extremely overweight (say about 25 kg or above your standard weight) or have bad knees, do not run, walk or do weight-bearing exercises, which cause strain and pain. Instead, go for 30 minutes stationary cycling. Various exercises that make a body flexible are described below:

Exercises for back, hips, thighs and buttocks

These ab-strengthening exercises take just ten minutes and can be done anywhere you find floor space. Apart from giving you a great shape, strong abdominal muscles are vital to your overall health and fitness. They take the strain off your back, aid digestion and can help relieve menstrual pain too.

○ Lie on the stomach with chin or forehead touching the ground. Stretch the arms to hold the folded legs. Raise upper part of the body as much as you can and also the legs as high as possible. Hold position for a few seconds. Repeat exercise three to four times. The exercise melts fat and has excellent effect on the muscles of shoulders, back, spine, hips, thighs, buttocks, waist and abdomen.

84

It leaves a beneficial effect on the digestive organs and cleanses the kidneys.

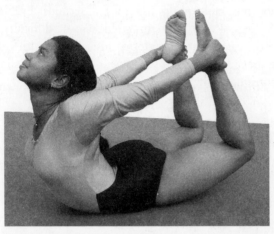

○ Lie on your back, palms on sides and heels together. Breathe normally. Now raise one leg upward slowly towards the sky in a perpendicular position, inhaling. Hold for 6-8 seconds and lower the leg towards floor, exhaling. Repeat exercise with other leg. Perform 4-5 rounds. This exercise is excellent to slim hips, thighs, buttocks, legs, waist and abdomen. It tones up the muscles of sex-glands, enhances potentiality, cures white vaginal discharge (leucorrhoea), menstrual disorders and aids digestive system.

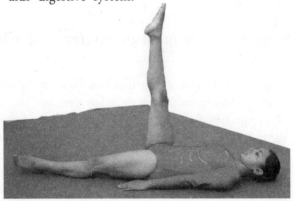

○ Lie on your stomach with chin touching the ground. Stretch arms on sides. Inhale. Raise legs as high as possible. Hold position for a few seconds. Exhale. Lower the legs. Repeat 3-4 times. In case of difficulty to raise both legs together, perform this exercise with one leg at a time, followed by the other. This exercise slims lower portion of the body.

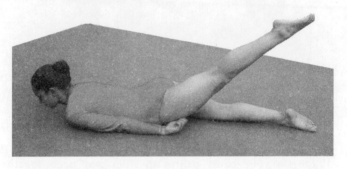

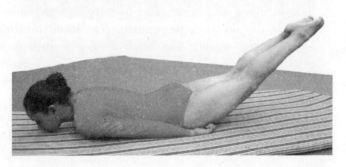

Gym helps to make back attractive and slim down hips

Do you know, men feel drawn to the back of a female, so make it as attractive as it can be. Here are a few exercises that can be performed at the health club to achieve desired result to make your back and hips attractive.

○ *Wide-grip pull downs exercise:* Sit or stand at the weight stack with your feet flat on the floor. Take a wide, overhand grip of the pull down bar with your hands wider than your shoulders. Start with your elbows slightly bent and pull the bar right to your chest. Do not swing or lean back as you pull the bar, but keep your back straight with a slight arch in the upper area. Control the weight through the complete movement and don't be afraid to use less weight. Do three sets of 8-10 repetitions.

○ *Close-grip pull downs exercise:* This movement targets the centre of the back region. Use the same technique as described above, moving your hands closer together. Don't lean back when you pull, instead remain upright when pulling the bar towards your chest. Do three sets of 8-10 repetitions.

○ *Bent-over barbell rows:* This exercise targets muscles of back, thighs, hips, rear shoulder and abdomen. Stand with knees slightly bent and back flat. Then bend at the hips until your torso is at an angle of 45 degrees. Grasp the barbell at shoulder width and hold your abdominal muscles tight to support your back. Pull it up to your chest, touching it to your ribs. Do three sets of 8-10 repetitions.

○ *Hips rotation exercise:* This exercise slims heavy hips. Stand on rotation equipment with straight back. Catch hold of bars and twist hips clockwise, anti-clockwise with heavy jerks. Repeat exercise until you feel a bit tired.

Mind-body fitness

Prepare for mind-body fitness. Experts do not advise instant weight loss, as health clubs and slimming centres usually claim. Instant weight-loss or inch-loss techniques harm the body. There is need of a strong, toned, slim and healthy mind-body. Here are some tips for mind-body fitness:

○ Right breathing and correct posture work wonders. Exercise with the right techniques.

○ Practice 15-20 minutes each for cardio and weight training programme daily.

87

- If you are making a weekly programme, keep three days for cardio, stretching and strengthening, and the remaining two days for weights.

- A casual walk after lunch or dinner should be a daily routine for everyone.

- Climb up the stairs after taking meals (except during periods, pregnancy and post-natal period). This helps to digest food.

- Be careful about cardio workouts, especially after general exercise routine or aerobics. The wrong twist or move could hurt you.

- If you are doing weights thrice a week, keep two days for the upper body (back, shoulders, chest and arms) and one for the lower body (calves, thighs and hips).

- An essential workout is a balanced mix of cardiovascular exercises, weight training and meditation.

- Always warm up prior to your workout even if you are in a hurry.

- Have water before a workout, sips in between and enough half an hour after the session.

- The floor where you are exercising has to be appropriate, preferably carpeted or soft wooden flooring. Concrete flooring will harm your joints.

- Wear the right footwear during workout.

- Eat well. It is vital to fitness. Cut down on fried foods, sweets and colas.

- Unless you don't get eight-hour sleep, you cannot aspire to fitness.

- Think positive, as a 100% ideal figure is never possible.

- Initially, exercise under a trained expert to avoid injury.

- Avoid jogging. You will have to pay its price later on after the age of 45 when you find weakness in joints and body strength. After this age we do not have the hormones that allow for increased muscle mass. Weights increase muscle tissues in the human body, which in turn cause weight gain.

○ Mind-body workout helps the bones, it is a powerful tool against osteoporosis. Beware of hurting yourself if you work without an instructor in a gym. Work with the right kind of equipment otherwise you might end up with problems of the lower back, spinal cord, elbow and shoulder joints.

○ Warm ups are important when working out with weights as well.

○ Don't ignore the spine. Stretching, strengthening and exercises are helpful to shape spine and strengthen spinal cord.

If you are over 60

If you are over sixty, choose simple warmth-inducing movements as following:

○ Try never to sit for longer than half an hour. Get up and do something—anything—and so keep your circulation on the go.

○ Sitting for a long time is harmful for muscles, joints, blood circulation and general feelings.

○ Don't sit about in a chair for a long time as this is very tiring. Better to walk about and then lie down again.

○ Do move about in bed and whenever you waken during the night, change your position.

○ When walking, see that the heels are level. Walk quickly across the floor using your ankles as fully as possible.

○ If you have to use a stick for any reason, don't let it slow you down. It should help you to keep as fast a stride as possible. It is just there to support you. If you are using stick, it should be carried in the hand opposite to the affected leg, never on the same side.

○ Never bend down over the stick, press on the handle. Beware of too big a stick, or you may damage your shoulder joint by pressure. Try always to have a stick with a curved handle so that you can hook it over your arm.

○ Every day, try to hurry enough at some time so that you become breathless for a minute or so.

○ Balancing on one leg is an excellent exercise.

Alternate methods of movement

Several methods of exercises and movement are described here briefly. There are many other kinds of exercise, dancing, physical training classes and visit to health clubs.

Aerobics

This method of exercise was devised in 1977 by Dr. Kenneth H. Cooper of the United States. Aerobics refers to a variety of activities like walking, jogging and running. The idea is to increase the maximum amount of oxygen that the body can process in given time. Aerobics builds basic fitness and endurance. It builds agility, co-ordination and muscular strength, particularly in the arms and upper torso.

Jogging

Jogging gives the necessary precautions, and explains how to take the pulse easily. Each jogger gets to know the reactions of his own body, mental, physical and emotional.

Yoga

Yoga originated in India and its roots are as ancient as Sanskrit. In Sanskrit, yoga means union or yoke. It means linking yourself to discipline through which you work towards balance and wholeness of body, mind and spirit. Yoga becomes a way of life, but we can choose what is useful for us and the physical postures or asanas are a good start.

Tai Chi Chuan, Karate and Judo

These are all forms of martial art which originated in China and Japan many centuries ago. They are still used widely as regimes for mind and body. Tai Chi Chuan consists in a variety of gentle continuous movements, which require control of the whole body and demand concentration, co-ordination and poise. All movements are circular, and develop balance and muscular control, rather than bulk.

Karate is a striking technique and Judo a grappling one. Judo has become very popular in the world amongst young people and has taken the place of boxing. It is an excellent form of exercise and can be very useful for self-defence. Judo is a strenuous exercise during which the pulse rate is likely to increase considerably and you sweat and breathe heavily. It works the whole body strongly – as you are moving yourself and another person is also trying to move you. Those suffering from high blood pressure and heart diseases should avoid practice of Tai Chi Chuan, Karate and Judo.

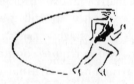

Chapter-9

Yoga Programme for Weight Loss

Obesity has become a worldwide health hazard and majority of people, male and female, of every age carry extra weight on their bodies, which not only develop physical disorders but also mental ailments, especially in women. Yoga has come to the rescue for obese persons. Regular practice of each and every yogic exercise affects and corrects some part of the body by melting extra fat. There are three categories of overweight: fatty overweight, watery overweight and cellulite, which have been described in separate chapters in this book.

Power Yoga or Ashtanga Yoga are the original postures designed by Patanjali, the sage who initiated yoga over 300 years ago. The word Ashtanga means eight-fold path: Ashta means eight and Anga means limbs. The eight limbs of yoga include:

○ Yama (ahinsa or non-violence), Satya (truth), Asetya (non-stealing), Brahmacharya (self-control) and Aparigraha (unselfishness).
○ Niyama, which refers to Saucha (cleanliness), Santosha (contentment)), Tapas (effort), Svadhyaya (self-study) and Ishwara Pranidhana (faith in God).
○ Asana means a posture.
○ Pranayama stands for control of the senses such as taste, touch, smell, sight and hearing.
○ Dharana means concentration.
○ Dhyana means meditation.
○ Samadhi means that unites with God.
○ And finally Yogasana.

What are Characteristics in obese persons

○ Usually addicted to overeating.

○ Habit of frequent eating.

○ Eat faster without chewing the food.

○ Retire soon after taking meal.

○ Not doing physical labour or exercise.

○ Daily intake of highly rich, high calorie foods.

○ Drinking lots of water with meals.

How to take care to avoid obesity

○ Take 10 to 12 glasses of fresh water in 24 hours.

○ Never eat more than 85% of your capacity at any time.

○ Drink water after ½ an hour of eating meal.

○ Naturopathy mentions integration of several ways to cure obesity such as vomation, laxative, taking enema for easy digestion, nasal wash for purification, intake of more water, sunbath, steam bath, fasting, habit of regular exercise, kunjal kriya, kati snan (hip bath), mud pack on abdomen and massage.

Why overweight

○ Intake of calorie-rich excessive diet resulting in deposition of fats in adipose cells.

○ Frequent eating.

○ Lack of exercise.

○ Eating freshly harvested cereals and excess meat.

○ Excessive intake of sweets.

○ Sleepiness during day time.

○ No sex.

○ No worry.

○ Happiness and hereditary factors.

○ When glucose contents of blood rise.

Symptoms

A person suffering from obesity may have one or more of the following symptoms:

- ○ Feeling of being hungry and thirsty.
- ○ Respiratory problem (half breathing).
- ○ Sleepiness.
- ○ More sweating.
- ○ Odour from the body.
- ○ Fatigue and heaviness.
- ○ Lack of enjoyment during sexual acts due to early exhaustion. The obese has less synthesis of semen and due to excessive deposition of fats in alimentary canal and the intestine, there is loss in their activity to a great extent.

Correcting obesity by Yoga

Yogic method of correcting obesity involves in taking a balanced and proper diet and practicing a few selected postures. It has been observed that an obese person loses an average 2 to 3 kg of weight per month by adopting above methods to fight obesity. Yogic method to reduce weight, though time consuming, is preferable and desirable due to the following reasons:

- ○ It reduces weight in a lasting and permanent way without causing any side effect to health, beauty and physical or mental condition.
- ○ It doesn't cost to correct obesity.
- ○ There is no disturbance to your normal life or a possibility of regaining the same weight even if yoga practice is discontinued.
- ○ Keep practicing yoga for 10 to 15 minutes daily although the weight has been reduced to normal level.
- ○ Continue yoga practice on selective basis. Initially, start with some of the selected easy-to-do postures for a week

94

or so, then proceed gradually but regularly, go on adding postures without any strain and exhaustion.

○ Start with simple warming up exercises before yoga practice. Rest for five minutes in Shavasana (in Sanskrit, shav means corpse) in the end of yoga session, which keeps mind and body relaxed. To practice *Shavasana*, lie on the back with arms at the sides, legs stretched out slightly apart. Close the eyes, breathe slowly and deeply relaxing each part, each muscle of the body, keeping brain completely empty. Avoid all mental stress, breathing rhythmically – inhaling and exhaling.

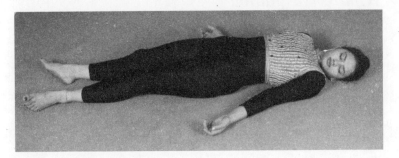

What is Pranayama

The Sanskrit word Prana means vital force or cosmic energy. Ayama means the control of the Prana, which signifies life or breath, and control of the vital force by concentration and regulated breathing. Breathing is essential to life: the absorption of air by the inhalation of oxygen and its expulsion by the exhalation of carbonic gas (carbon dioxide). The yogic breathing consists of three parts as explained below. Always inhale and exhale through the nose.

○ The abdomen: Inhale and allow the abdomen to expand like a bow. The lungs fill with air during exhalation. This is an excellent exercise for abdomen, which regularises the functioning of the intestines and stimulates digestion.

- The middle part of the chest (thorax): Put the hands on either side of the ribs. Inhale slowly inflating the sides thoroughly, then exhale and repeat several times. The process purifies blood, improves circulation and calms the heart.
- The upper part of the chest or collar bones (clavicle): Put hands on each side of clavicle. Contract the stomach slightly. Inhale slowly pushing the clavicle upwards, then begin to exhale pushing it downwards. Repeat several times. The process cleans and fortifies the upper chest.

What is Meditation

The posture develops physical and mental stability, calms the nerves, relieves stiffness of the joints, supplies blood to abdominal region and the entire body is kept in complete equilibrium. *Padmasana* is a meditation posture. To practice this posture, begin by placing the right foot on the left thigh and then left foot on the right thigh. The hands are kept open resting on the knees. Keep the head and spinal column straight.

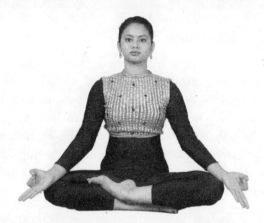

Rules to practice Pranayama or Yoga

- Start practice not before the age of eight to ten years.
- Yoga exercise is equally useful for both sexes: male and female.

- ○ Always practice in a peaceful, calm, noiseless and airy environment.
- ○ Wear clothes which are sufficient to protect the body.
- ○ Avoid wearing tight clothes.
- ○ Practice on empty stomach, two hours after breakfast and four hours after a meal, and an hour after having a cup of tea or coffee.
- ○ Start practicing for short periods and gradually increase the duration.
- ○ The practitioner should be a vegetarian as far as possible.

Useful tips for practicing Yoga

- ○ Warming up exercise is essential before yoga practice for slimming, shaping figure and obtaining perfect results.
- ○ Brisk walk in the fresh morning air is very beneficial and gives exercise to the whole body, especially useful for hips and thighs.
- ○ Always cool down after a yoga session. You begin to feel more poised, loose limbed, coordinated, stretched and toned, feel as if you are gliding rather than walking.
- ○ If you are overweight (about 20 kg or above your standard weight) do not run. Remember, weight-bearing exercises strain your joints even more.
- ○ Pre-exercise meal should be light.
- ○ Cool down after exercising a session with slow and gentle stretches.
- ○ Consult a doctor or a yoga teacher before embarking on any yogic exercise program, especially when you are above 45 years of age, pregnant, have a personal or family history of high blood pressure or heart problem.
- ○ Too much and too fast yogic practice does not provide instant results; these simply lead to injuries, aches and pains.

What is Power Yoga

It is a combination of dynamic breathing, strong flowing movement that creates a high-heat, high-energy workout. Yoga helps flow of energy into the body, builds strength, releases tension from joints and cleanses the body of toxins. Don't overdo yoga exercises else you could put undue strain on your muscles and joints. The exercise must be done under the guidance of a qualified yoga teacher. Teenagers, especially girls between the age of 14 and 18 tend to put on excess weight largely because their bodies undergo natural changes around this time. Women usually face this problem after delivering their first baby. Obesity is disastrous for women and it becomes a real mental burden for those afflicted with it. Although the problem does not cause physical harm to the health, its psychological effect can be far more damaging for figure-conscious women. You may control overweight without tears by practicing yogic exercises regularly. To maintain a perfect figure, the amount of energy you consume must be equal to the amount of energy you burn.

Surya Namaskar Asana (sun exercise)

This is the most recommended yogic exercise to fight overweight and stimulate the muscles of the whole body. This asana involves various bending forward and backward movements. The regular practice of Surya Namaskar asana helps to stretch and strengthen all major muscles of the body, improve blood circulation to the organs, replenishing them with fresh oxygen and nutrients, strengthen the upper and lower body and abdominal muscles, thereby making it a complete fitness routine. The posture has twelve positions as described below:

○ **Position 1:** Stand facing the direction of the Sun with your weight evenly distributed and your back straight. Exhale as you put your palms together in the 'prayer pose'.

○ **Position 2:** Inhale as you stretch your arms back above the head so that your back arches and your head is tilted back.

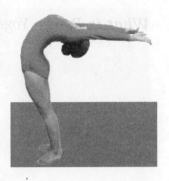

○ **Position 3:** Exhale slowly bending forward, touching the earth with respect until the hands are in line with the feet, head touching the knees.

○ **Position 4:** Inhale as you extend your left leg behind you, resting the knee on the ground. Raise the head.

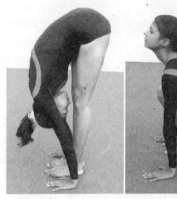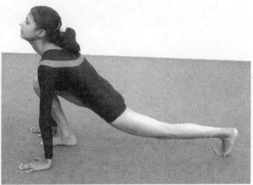

○ **Position 5:** Exhale as you extend your right leg too and hold your breath as you push yourself up on your feet. Raise your hips so that your body forms an inverted 'V'.

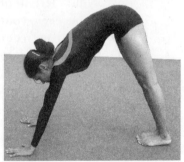

○ **Position 6:** Exhale as you lower your knees, chest and chin on the floor. The hips are off the floor.

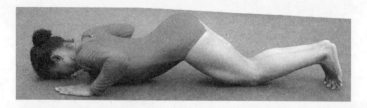

○ **Position 7:** Inhale and slowly raise head, trunk, hips, thighs and knees from floor, keeping backwards.

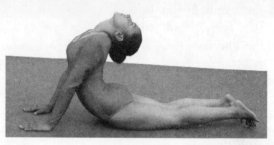

○ **Position 8:** While exhaling, bring the left foot together with the right. Keep arms straight. Raise your hips and form an inverted 'V'.

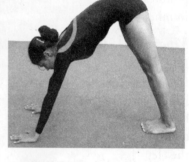

○ **Position 9:** Inhale as you move your left foot forward between your hands, allowing your right knee to bend to the floor, and look up. Left leg remains stretched.

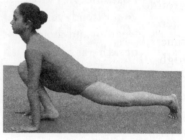

○ **Position 10:** Raise the body with hands backward.

○ **Position 11:** Bend backward with raised hands and feet joined.

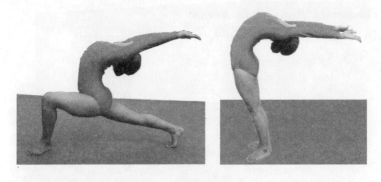

○ **Position 12:** Return to the original standing position with folded hands.

Postures to stimulate muscles of face and upper portion of body

Viparitakarani and Parasarita Pada-uttan are recommended yogic postures for enhancing the beauty of face and prevent fat from forming on the upper portion of body.

Viparitakarani Asana (inverted posture)

In Sanskrit, Viparita means inverted and karani means action. Lie on the back. Inhale. Raise legs and hips with the help of hands/arms. Exhale. The legs should form an angle of 60-70 degrees. Lower the legs gently on the ground. Relax. Repeat exercise three to four times. If you suffer from high blood pressure, consult a doctor before doing this posture. This posture is beneficial for

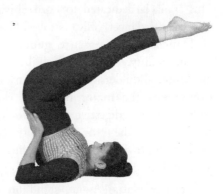

reviving the body and prevents formation of facial wrinkles. The posture also regenerates thyroid and pituitary glands, controls nervous system and increases flow of blood to neck, throat and head.

101

Parasarita Pada-uttan Asana

To do this posture, following steps are undertaken:

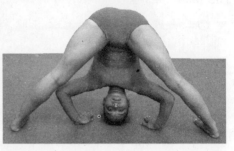

- ○ Spread your legs about three feet apart.
- ○ Place palms on the floor and also rest crown of your head on the floor.
- ○ Remain in this position for 15 to 20 seconds, then raise your head and jump in standing position.
- ○ Repeat this asana 3-4 times.

This exercise not only increases the beauty of face and upper portion of body but also removes fatigue, relieves aches and cramps in the calf muscles, helps hair growth and strengthens the muscles of back, hips and thighs.

How to slim hips and thighs

Natraj Asana

This asana is dedicated to Lord Shiva. As a cosmic dancer, Shiva is called God of Dances. This posture generates vigour, vitality, potency, flexibility to the limbs, shoulders and hip joints. It strengthens the major bones of the body, enhances digestive power, leaves good effect on the spine, removes spinal rigidity, improves eyesight, slims heavy hips and thighs,

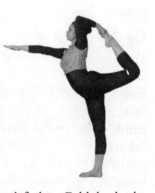

To practice Natraj Asana, stand on the left leg. Fold back the right leg at the knee and grab toes of the right leg with the palm of right hand folding the right leg backwards. Stay in this position for 8-10 seconds and keep breathing normal. Now repeat the whole posture on other foot. Make four to six rounds daily.

Trikon Asana (triangle posture)

This posture prevents formation of fat around hips and thighs. The following steps are recommended to do this exercise:

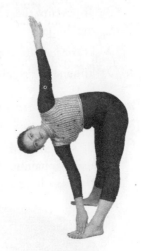

- ◯ Stand with legs apart. Inhale. Raise the arm.
- ◯ Rotate waist and begin to exhale until the fingers of the right hand touch the ground. The arms should form a vertical line with the face turned upwards.
- ◯ Stand up inhaling at the same time. Perform the same movement with other hand.
- ◯ Finish the exercise by exhaling.

How to slim your back

Yog Mudra and Paschimottan Asana are recommended postures to strengthen back muscles and also to remove extra fat from thighs and hips.

Yog Mudra

Also known as 'the symbol of yoga'. Sit in the Padmasana position keeping the spinal column upright. Place hands behind the back and grab the wrist of one hand with the other hand. Inhale. Now lean forward gently and slowly without straining or jerking the spinal column, exhaling, until the forehead touches the floor. Stay in this position as long as you feel comfortable without breathing.

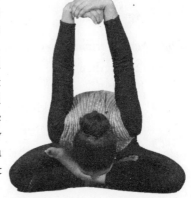

Therapeutic advantages of this asana include the following:

- Dissolves fat deposits from back, hips and thighs.
- Remedy for constipation and digestive system.
- Tones up the abdominal muscles/organs and exercises the lungs.
- Leaves curative effect for asthma patients.
- Enhances sexual potentiality.

Paschimottan Asana (stretching the back and legs)

To do this asana:

- Sit straight with feet together. Raise the arms above the head, inhaling. Lean forward exhaling until the head touches the knees, which should remain flat.

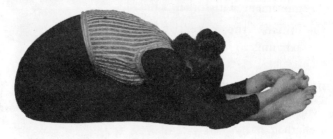

- Hold the big toe of right foot with the thumb and index finger of the left hand. Inhale and stay in this position for seven seconds.
- Then gradually sit up. Exhale and relax. Repeat exercise for 3-4 times.

Therapeutic advantages of this posture include the following:

- Strengthens the muscles of back, abdomen and spinal column.
- It regenerates kidneys and digestive organs. Cures diabetes and constipation.
- Prevents formation of fat around the stomach and back.
- It helps blood to flow to the gonads, prostate glands, uterus and bladder.

Yoga postures to relieve fat on stomach, waist and trunk

Hal Asana (plough posture)

To do this asana, following steps are recommended:

- ○ Lie on the back, arms stretched by the side.
- ○ Raise legs slowly, stretched vertically.
- ○ Then lower the legs behind the head until the tips of the feet touch the ground.

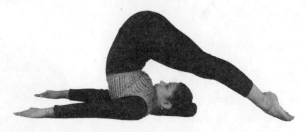

- ○ Remain in this position for 25-40 seconds breathing regularly.
- ○ Return to the starting position. Relax and repeat the posture four to five times.

Besides relieving fatness on stomach, waist and trunk, this posture helps relieve digestive problems, increases supply of blood to facial muscles and head, has regenerating effect on the glandular system, clears menstrual disorders and removes exhaustion and fatigue.

Vajroli Mudra (boat posture)

This balancing pose strengthens stomach, waist, thighs, hips and abdominal muscles. The asana rids the digestive organs of toxins and helps to develop the sexual will power in women between the ages of 20 to 40 years.

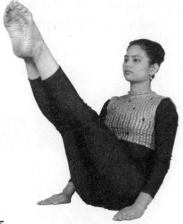

Janusir Asana, Parivritta Janusir Asana and Janusir Merudanda Asana

These yoga postures are especially beneficial for women to eradicate wrinkles on the waist, lower abdomen and fat around

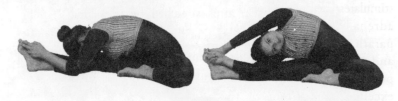

hips, thighs, buttocks and legs after childbirth. Janusir Asana (head touching knee position) involves placing the foot of the bent leg on the thighs of the other leg. In Parivritta Janusir Asana (head-to-toe position), the foot of the leg lying flat is touched by the hands with the body leaning to one side. This posture also tones up the muscles of spinal column besides removing excess fat around the waist, hips and abdomen. Janusir Merudanda Asana (head, knee and spinal column posture) has similar benefits as in case

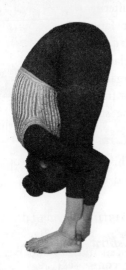

of above and cures disorders of menstruation, strengthens genital (reproductive) organs among women after childbirth.

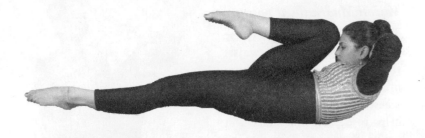

Postures to slim abdomen and spine
Dhanur Asana (the bow posture)

This yoga posture not only tones up the abdominal organs, it loosens up the spinal column, strengthens the nervous centres, stimulates the endocrine adrenal, the thyroid, parathyroid, pituitary and sex glands. The practice of this asana is excellent for women suffering from irregular or faulty menstruation and other troubles related to reproductive organs. It also prevents fat from forming around the stomach, waist and hips.

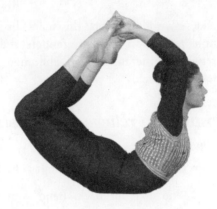

Kurm Asana (the tortoise posture)

This yogic posture has a beneficial effect on the spinal column and tones up abdominal organs, which are charged with energy.

Posture for slimming legs, knees and ankles
Ushtra Asana (the camel posture)

It comprises the following steps:

- ◯ Fold the legs at the knees keeping them six inches apart.
- ◯ Rest your hands on hips.
- ◯ Stand on knees and let the ankles and toes of the both legs fall flat on the floor.

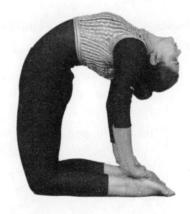

- ○ Curve back and catch hold of the soles of your feet.
- ○ After 10 to 15 counts return to initial position bringing one hand at a time.
- ○ Repeat this posture 2 to 4 times.

Besides slimming down, this asana brings good effect upon the whole respiratory system, renders the spinal column flexible, strengthens the muscles of abdomen, spine, thighs, buttocks, chest and arms.

Postures to relieve spinal column deformities

Sarvang Asana

To do this asana, the following steps are advised:

- ○ Lie on your back. Bend your knees towards the chest.
- ○ Raise your hips and legs off the floor supporting back with your palms.
- ○ Straighten your legs perpendicular to the floor.

This asana helps relieve headaches, cold, cough, constipation, enhances facial beauty and improves functioning of all organs, glands and nerves of face and upper part of body.

Bhujang Asana (cobra posture)

This is most beneficial for spinal column.

- ○ Lie on your stomach, joining legs. Place your palms to the sides of your breasts.
- ○ Inhale. Supporting the arms, slowly raise your head and trunk leaning backwards as far as possible without raising the abdominal region from the ground.

108

○ Hold this position for a few seconds. Exhale. Slowly and gradually return to starting position.

○ Repeat the exercise three to four times.

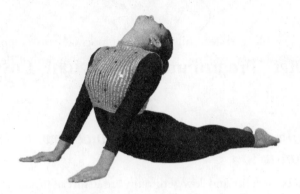

Therapeutic advantages

○ Supplies blood to spinal column region.

○ Strengthens the muscles of breasts.

○ Enhances facial beauty.

○ Avoids double chin.

○ Leaves beneficial effect on the kidneys (adrenal glands) and stimulates digestion.

○ Cures constipation, indigestion, dysentery, wind troubles and abdominal disorders.

○ Has specific benefits for women and corrects various menstrual problems.

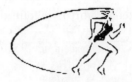

Chapter-10

Diet Programme for Weight Loss

Do calorie-restriction diets induce low serotonin

The excess insulin and low serotonin are a threat to good health and getting obese. Good calories prevent both of these from developing. You need a calorie-restriction programme if you want to lose less than 7 kg. and have normal insulin level. Eating serotonin-stimulating foods transforms calorie restriction by an easy-to-follow programme because it doesn't cause you to suffer from the food cravings, depression and low serotonin irritability. You will be in a position to lose weight faster than with a conventional calorie-restriction programme. Clinical study reveals, the effectiveness of good calories has shown increased rate of weight loss. Make sure to be very careful about eating good calories, otherwise you may find your serotonin chemistry harmful, and for losing a few kilos of weight you may have to pay a high price.

What is the effect of serotonin on weight loss

A woman has to eat food to sustain her serotonin chemistry. Weight-loss diet has been designed for both male and female body. Remember, all conventional diets lower a woman's serotonin. High-protein, low fat and high-carbohydrate diets all bring on abnormal serotonin. It has been observed that even conventional serotonin-boosting diets fail to meet a woman's need and may lower serotonin.

However, there are several serotonin-stimulating drugs (such as Prozac, Redux or Fenaflurmine), but such drugs carry the risk of very harmful side effects and should not be taken without consulting a doctor. Women with low serotonin are seen often suffering from a sense of panic, anxiety, stress and depression. It affects every woman differently. Symptoms of low serotonin include the following:

O Weight gain
O Depression
O Stress
O Tendency toward substance abuse
O Pre-menstrual stress
O Food cravings and eating disorders
O Sexual dysfunction
O Anxiety
O Irritability
O Disturbed sleep (insomnia)
O Frequent headaches
O Obsessive and compulsive behaviour
O Inability to form proper social relationship
O Lower social dominance

There are two diet programmes that support a woman's serotonin, increase her well-being and allow her to lose weight easily.

1. Serotonin and a woman's psyche

Women need different food as their brains have much more serotonin than men because of higher storage capacity as female sex hormones enhance serotonin activity. A woman's higher levels of serotonin may be of fundamental importance for functions such as appetite, sexuality, impulsive behaviour, cooperative attitude and aggression.

2. Supporting a woman's serotonin

Women need to eat serotonin-stimulating foods that support serotonin synthesis. In the absence of these foods, the serotonin levels will decrease affecting a woman's brain. Good calorie diets elevate mood, banish food cravings, lift depression, make sex enjoyable and help weight loss in women.

When you don't lose weight on the free-eating plan

If you fail to lose weight on the free-eating programme, you must question yourself: "Am I following the programme correctly?" The following are some of the most common reasons that dieters deprive themselves of benefits:

1. Eating a breakfast of low-protein; good calorie carbohydrates.
2. Eating too much animal protein.
3. Combining protein or saturated fats with starches.
4. Snacking on bad calories.
5. Skipping meals very often.
6. Eating too much saturated fat.
7. Eating too little unsaturated fat.
8. Eating too late at night.

How to relieve stress

Stressed women excrete essential vitamins and minerals. It is very important to keep insulin levels under control. When insulin levels become out of control, stressed women are more susceptible to the food addiction. Prolactin is a hormone released during mental or physical stress. When dieting, a woman's prolactin rises by more than 50% whereas a man's prolactin remains unchanged. Dieting creates stress in women and sometimes it creates conditions that can lead to food addiction. Dieting women have a special need to reduce stress. There are three techniques for lowering stress: *Exercise, Meditation and Breathing*. Reducing stress is a powerful tool to boost your physical and mental health, which makes weight loss easier.

Exercise

Most weight loss programmes recommend exercise a means to burn excess calories. Many of such programmes fail due to unbalanced plan disturbing the functioning of serotonin and insulin. Never overdo exercise. Many dieting women harm their bodies with such a fury of exercise resulting in prolactin, serotonin, and other important hormones going into the stress mode. All you need is 30 minutes of exercise every day. You can do more, but only if you gradually build up to a higher level. Remember: Over-exercising is Harmful. The following guidelines are suggested:

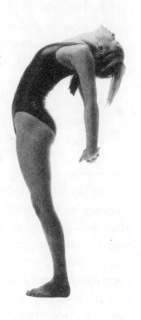

1. Find an exercise you enjoy.
2. Exercise for at least 30 minutes, five times per week.
3. Never exercise to exhaustion.

"What type of exercise should be adopted?" dieting women usually ask this question. Repetitive muscle movements are most effective at elevating serotonin. Walking, jogging, cycling, swimming, aerobics, climbing stairs and running are highly recommended forms of exercise. Ancient Hatha Yoga and Tai Chi are also excellent forms of exercise for overweight persons. These ancient disciplines are based on a balanced approach to fitness, especially useful for the entire mind-body connection. These forms of exercise make you feel energised, calm and revitalised. The best form of exercise for a housewife to maintain her body is one that you must do: walking, jogging, gardening, playing golf, dancing and doing anything that gets you moving.

Meditation

It is the ultimate way to reduce stress with the following effects:

○ To lower heart rate and blood pressure.

○ Reduce the hormones associated with stress, prolactin and glucocorticoids.

○ Counter a dieting woman's tendency toward depression and low serotonin.

○ Lower the thyroid-stimulating hormones, which create depression.

○ Increase serotonin activity.

The beginners usually ask a question: "What is meditation and how to do it?" Meditation is concentration of mind, which is necessary to accomplish anything in life. If you don't concentrate when you drive, your vehicle will indulge into a mishap on the road. Concentration is necessary when studying. If you don't concentrate on your work, you will not be productive. In fact, concentration is the continued flow of our attention to an object or activity. You will like to know the difference between concentration and meditation. Concentration is externally directed, whereas meditation is directed to one's inner self. Breathing and mantras are tools to help us to meditate while sitting in a posture anytime, anywhere.

What is Mantra

A *mantra* is a phase to help you enter meditation easily. There is strong connection between meditation and mantra. Simply repeating the mantra silently lets you immediately enter into a more meditative awareness.'*Hamsa mantra*' is extremely powerful and as simple as listening to your breath. If you listen closely while breathing, you can hear its subtle sound – Hamsa. 'Ham' (pronounced hamm) is the sound when inhaling whereas 'Sa' (pronounced saahh) is the sound of the outgoing breath. *Hamsa is the actual vibrational sound of one's inner self.* Observing your breath in this way leads to relaxation. When changing breathing pattern one changes his/her emotional state as explained.

Mood	Pattern of breathing
When angry	Holding breath and taking deep gulps of air.
When nervous or afraid	Rapid and shallow breathing.
When relaxed	Long, deep breathing.
When calm	Deep and slow breathing.

Your breath mirrors your thoughts and emotions. If you don't want to use Hamsa mantra, you can simply focus on your breath, which can give you an enormous boost of energy and mental clarity. The way you breathe during meditation is the way you naturally breathe when you are calm: slowly, evenly and deeply. Breathing this way makes your mind receptive to meditation. Following are correct meditation techniques:

○ Breathe deeply.

○ Coordinate mantra with the rhythm of your breathing.

○ As you inhale, silently repeat 'ham'.

○ As you exhale, silently repeat 'sa'.

○ Hear these sounds in your breath.

○ You are ready to start regular meditation sessions.

The following precautions are taken when meditating:

○ Meditate at the same time every day – early morning, late evening or before going to bed when the surrounding is quieter.

○ Whatever time you choose, try to be regular.

○ Sit at the same place daily.

○ Meditate in a quiet room. If you don't have that luxury just find a quiet corner and make it your meditative haven.

○ Begin with 15 minutes.

○ Sit comfortably on the floor with your legs crossed, in a relaxed, comfortable, upright position.

- O Keep your back and neck straight, without stiffening your muscles, to allow full, deep breathing.
- O Meditation should provide you the ability to experience the calm that lies beyond the mind.

Harmful effect of modern diet on serotonin system

Usually modern diet is very high in protein and high-sugar foods. Nearly every meal contains meat, fish, poultry or dairy protein. Most of the modern diet consists of baked goods, candy and processed foods, which are high in sugar. But these foods leave a harmful effect on woman's serotonin. In ancient times, fruits and vegetables had less sugar content than today's varieties. Many modern women eat diets high in protein and full of high sugar foods, and those neglecting their diet may become overweight, can go through life impaired by low serotonin. In fact, such problems have become just part of being a woman. Low serotonin causes constant state of stress brought on by fighting negative impulses. It is not possible to function properly under stress, resulting in loss of control of mind and being emotional and more prone to negative thoughts.

Problems associated with low serotonin

Food cravings and depression are two main afflictions controlled by serotonin that often plague a woman's mind. Modern food brings on low serotonin levels and impairs women, so they do not have the emotional and mental energy. Modern foods and weight loss diets make women become emotional, depressed, fatigued and prone to extreme behaviours. On the other hand, men do not suffer from these problems.

- O **Impaired social interactions:** Serotonin has been linked to the formation of social groups, grooming, maintaining social proximity and other forms of social cooperative behaviour.

O **Appropriate behaviour:** Serotonin helps us avoid unpleasant situations by controlling memories.

O **Excessive behaviour:** Serotonin is necessary to stop impulsive (aggressive, violent and destructive) behaviour. Informations reveal, 80% women committing suicide were found suffering from low levels of serotonin.

O **Menopause:** During menopause the hormones that elevate serotonin decrease, which tend to impair serotonin synthesis. Many psychological sysmptoms of menopause are due to changes in serotonin. That is why women gain weight during menopause.

O **Obsessive-compulsive disorder:** Such persons exhibit an abnormally high degree of fear, doubt, anxiety and a need to control their environment. Common obsessions include sexual obsession, aggressive behaviour, excessive fear of failure and the need for sympathy.

O **Overeating after stopping smoking:** Such persons may suffer from symptoms, especially carbohydrate cravings, which are consistent with low serotonin levels.

O **Sexuality:** Low serotonin makes it difficult for women to be sexually receptive. High serotonin inhibits a man's sexual drive. It stimulates a woman's sexual responsiveness.

O **Sleep disturbance:** Sleeplessness is linked to low serotonin.

O **Premenstrual stress:** Serotonin levels rise and fall during the menstrual cycle, reaching their lowest point just before the start of menstruation and at the time when menstruation is at the peak.

O Other conditions due to low levels of serotonin include the following:

1. Arthritis
2. Bipolar disorders
3. Unstable mood and behaviour

4. Extreme muscle weakness (cataplexy)
5. Chronic pain
6. Chronic low-grade depression (dysthymia)
7. Emotional liability
8. Hyperactivity
9. Hypochondria
10. Hypomania (abnormal mood elevation)
11. Panic disorder
12. Post-traumatic stress syndrome
13. Schizophrenia
14. Winter depression (seasonal affective disorder)
15. Self-injurious behaviour
16. Social phobia

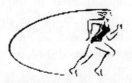

Diet and Nutrition Programme

Different methods of cooking

The following effects on the nutrients in foods due to cooking have been registered:

1. Cooking by water causes loss of vitamin C. Between 30 to 70% water-soluble vitamins and minerals are lost.

2. Cooking by steam causes loss of vitamin C and a few other vitamins.

3. Cooking in pressure cooker results in moderate loss of vitamin C and slight loss of vitamin B12.

4. Deep frying results in destruction of thiamin, vitamin A, carotene and vitamin C.

5. Shallow frying causes moderate loss of vitamin C and slight loss of vitamin A, carotene and thiamin.

6. Dry roasting leads to heavy loss of thiamin and reduces nutritive value of protein.

7. Cooking soda added to food causes 70% loss of thiamin and 30% of riboflavin.

7. Sprouting of pulse increases vitamin C content and also the digestibility.

Cooking has several advantages. It improves the palatability, quality and digestibility of food.

Vegetarianism vs. non-vegetarianism

Non-vegetarian food is considered an important factor in daily diet due to the presence of complete protein, which causes heavy work to the kidneys and lessens the efficiency of the organs leading to degenerative disorders.

○ Death rate among non-vegetarians by coronary heart disease has been recorded higher as compared to the vegetarians because of higher levels of cholesterol and fat absorbed into the system through non-vegetarian diet.

○ Non-vegetarian food adds calories and leads to obesity, diabetes and high blood pressure.

○ The tissues of all animals contain poisonous wastes. When non-vegetable food is consumed, toxic level in the system increases. Soya bean is a better substitute to meat.

○ Non-vegetarian food products stored in cold storage when reheated result in rapid decomposition since the non-vegetarian diet is relatively low in fibre content.

○ The movement of food in bowels slows down resulting in exposure to the large intestine. The toxins present in the non-vegetarian food lead to risk of colon cancer.

○ A well-selected vegetable diet can supply good quality protein and such food definitely is superior to the non-vegetable diet.

Nutritional value of foods we eat

○ **Coffee:** Caffeine present in the coffee stimulates the adrenal gland to release into blood stream raising the blood pressure, blood sugar, pulse and heart rates. A cup of coffee contains up to 100 mg of caffeine. Most common problems faced by coffee consumers are insomnia, slightly raised blood pressure and inability to relax.

○ **Tea:** Contains toxin (caffeine).

○ **Colas and chocolates:** These contain caffeine and have to be strictly avoided during dieting period. They cause health problems and interfere in the detoxification and cleansing process in the body.

O **Alcohol:** Alcoholic drinks lead to severe addiction and raise tryglyceride (a type of fat) levels in the blood. 1 gm of alcohol yields 7 calories and 1 gm of fat yields 9 calories. Excessive alcohol drinking leads to alcohol dependency, obesity, vitamin B deficiency, high blood pressure, increased tendency to stroke and paralysis, liver damage and it tranquillises the brain, which may cause accidents.

Fruits and vegetables that check obesity and add glamour

Apple	Carbohydrate present in the apple helps in stimulation and peristalsis and relieves constipation. Apple reduces cholesterol and is antioxidant.
Amla	Rich in pectin and vitamin C. It's cooling, diuretic and laxative in nature.
Banana	Contains appreciable amount of vitamins (A,B,C and D), calcium, magnesium, phosphorus, iron and copper.
Figs	Contains high sugar content. It relieves constipation.
Grapes	A revitalising fruit, which contains ample protein, carbohydrates, vitamin A and B and minerals. It helps in elimination of toxins from the system and purifies blood.
Grapefruit	A citrus fruit rich in potassium, vitamin A and vitamin B.
Guava	Very rich in vitamin C and regulates bowel movement.
Lemon	A citrus fruit, rich in citric acid and alkaline. After complete digestion vitamin C in the lemon juice strengthens connective tissues of

121

the joints, improves the vitality and is useful in treating colds and coughs.

Mango	It's rich in vitamin A and C. It cures diabetes and obesity.
Water melon	Being low in calories, it is ideal for weight watchers. It's cooling, refreshing and rich in vitamin C.
Musk melon	It's rich in alkaline salt. Treats hyperacidity, ulcers and other digestive disorders.
Orange	Rich in vitamin A,B,C and calcium. It is digestive and an excellent blood purifier.
Papaya	A highly alkaline and digestive fruit. Rich in vitamin A,B,C and D.
Pomegranate	It's rich in sugar, iron and citric acid. Relieves constipation and prevent diarrhoea.
Pineapple	Helps in digestion. Pineapple juice contains a substance almost similar to pepsin present in stomach. It raises alkalinity and purifies blood.
Pear	Contains more sugar and less acid. It is useful in case of bladder stone.
Sapota (chiku)	A high calorie fruit; hence diabetics and those having obesity should avoid. It is useful in relieving constipation.
Vegetables	These are consumed in the form of leaf, stem, root and flower. They are either used raw or after cooking. Root and tuber vegetables are rich in carbohydrates, low in fat and protein. Important root and tuber vegetables are beetroot, carrot, potato, sweet potato, radish, turnip, onion, garlic, ginger, etc.
Beetroot	It's juicy and rich in alkaline salts. It is a good source of potassium, sodium, magnesium and iron.
Radish	Very low calorie vegetable and has diuretic effect.

Turnip	A rich source of calcium having juicy root vegetable with pungent flavour.
Carrot	A rich source of vitamin A. Helps in case of anaemia. It is a blood purifier. Carrot juice is very useful for asthmatics, hyperacidity patients, under-nourished people, and treating ulcers.
Potato	A good source of vitamin C. It contains starch and is alkaline. Consists of approx. 70% moisture, 20% carbohydrates, 2% protein and minerals (potassium and magnesium).
Onion	It is classified under spice category and also has medical value. It reduces cholesterol levels and is a powerful antiseptic.
	Has remarkable curative properties, which help to bring down cholesterol and release flatulence/ gas from the stomach.
Ginger	Contains 80% moisture, little amount of protein and fibre. It is also carminative, stimulant, blood purifier and stimulates appetite.

Some dietary do's and don'ts

○ Excessive use of fruits and raw vegetables is useful. Carrots, radish, lettuce, spinach, cauliflower and cabbage are useful vegetables.

○ Use whole wheat such as brown bread, chapaties, etc.

○ Use plenty of fibrous food such as beans, bran, leafy vegetables, oat flakes, China grass, isabgol, etc.

○ Intake of liquids such as water, lemon juice, fruit juices, etc. rids toxins from the body.

○ Use of confectioneries, pastries, cakes, sweets, etc. should be curtailed.

○ All dry fruits, figs, prunes, raisins, apricot and plums have laxative effect. Fresh fruits such as grapes, figs, papaya, banana, mango and orange should be encouraged.

○ Taking 2 to 4 glasses of water immediately after getting up from bed stimulates bowel movement.

○ Soak dry fruits such as raisins, dates in milk or plain water and taking it before going to bed at night or in the morning is very useful in the treatment of constipation.

○ Taking 2-3 teaspoons of 'isabgol' with milk or warm water either at bedtime or early in the morning is very useful.

1800 calorie vegetarian menu

Meal	Menu	Weight	Measure
Breakfast	Bread	60 gm	3 slices
	Milk	140 ml	1 cup
	Fruit	100 gm	1 no.
	Butter	6.3 gm	1 tsp
Mid morning snack	Biscuits	10 gm	2 no.
	Fruit	100 gm	1 no.
Lunch	3 Chapaties or		
	Cooked rice	75 gm (raw)	
	Daal	25 gm (raw)	1 katori
	Curds	75 gm	½ katori
	Assorted vegetables		1½ katori
	Cooking oil	10 gm	2 tsp
Tea	Biscuits	10 gm	2 no.
	Fruit	100 gm	1 no.
Dinner	3 Chapaties or		
	Cooked rice	75 gm (raw)	
	Daal	75 gm	1 katori
	Curds	75 gm	½ katori
	Assorted vegetables		1½ katori
	Cooking oil	10 gm	
Bedtime	Milk	140 ml	1 cup

124

1800 calorie non-vegetarian menu

Meal	Menu	Weight	Measure
Breakfast	Bread	80 gm	4 slices
	Milk	140 ml	1 cup
	Butter	6.3 gm	1 tsp
Mid morning snack	Biscuits	10 gm	2 no.
	Fruit	100 gm	1 no.
Lunch	4 Chapaties or		
	Cooked rice	100 gm	
	Daal	25 gm	1 katori
	Curds	75 gm	½ katori
	Assorted vegetables		1½ katori
	Cooking oil	10 gm	2 tsp
Tea	Biscuits	20 gm	4 no.
	Fruit	100 gm	1 no.
Dinner	3 Chapaties or		
	Cooked rice	75 gm	
	Meat/Fish		
	Assorted vegetables		1½ katori
	Cooking oil	10 gm	2 tsp
Bedtime	Milk	70 ml	½ cup

2000 calorie vegetarian menu

Meal	Menu	Weight	Measure
Breakfast	Bread	80 gm	4 slices
	Milk	140 ml	1 cup
	Fruit	100 gm	1 no.
	Butter	12.6 gm	2 tsp
Mid morning snack	Biscuits	10 gm	2 no.
	Fruit	100 gm	1 no.
Lunch	4 Chapaties or		
	Cooked rice	100 gm	
	Daal	25 gm	1 katori
	Curds	140 gm	1 katori

125

	Assorted vegetables		2 katories
	Cooking oil	10 gm	2 tsp
Tea	Biscuits	10 gm	2 no.
	Fruit	100 gm	1 no.
Dinner	3 Chapaties or		
	Cooked rice	75 gm	
	Daal	75 gm	1 katori
	Curds	75 gm	½ katori
	Assorted vegetables		1½ katori
	Cooking oil	10 gm	2 tsp
Bedtime	Milk	140 ml	1 cup

2000 calories non-vegetarian menu

Meal	*Menu*	*Weight*	*Measure*
Breakfast	Bread	80 gm	4 slices
	Milk	140 ml	1 cup
	Butter	6.3 gm	1 tsp
Mid morning snack	Biscuits	10 gm	2 no.
	Fruit	100 gm	1 no.
Lunch	4 Chapaties or		
	Cooked rice	100 gm	
	Daal	25 gm	1 katori
	Curds	75 gm	½ katori
	Assorted vegetables		2 katories
	Cooking oil	15 gm	3 tsp
Tea	Biscuits	20 gm	4 no.
	Fruit	100 gm	1 no.
Dinner	4 Chapaties or		
	Cooked rice	75 gm	
	Meat/Fish		
	Assorted vegetables		1½ katori
	Cooking oil	15 gm	3 tsp
Bedtime	Milk	70 ml	½ cup

2200 calorie vegetarian meal

Meal	Menu	Weight	Measure
Breakfast	Bread	80 gm	4 slices
	Milk	140 ml	1 cup
	Fruit	100 gm	1 no.
	Butter	12.6 gm	2 tsp
Mid morning snack	Biscuits	10 gm	2 no.
	Fruit	100 gm	1 no.
Lunch	4 Chapaties or		
	Cooked rice	100 gm	
	Daal	25 gm	1 katori
	Curds	140 gm	1 katori
	Assorted vegetables		2 katories
	Cooking oil	15 gm	3 tsp
Tea	Biscuits	20 gm	4 no.
	Fruit	100 gm	1 no.
Dinner	3 Chapaties or		
	Cooked rice	100 gm	
	Daal	25 gm	1 katori
	Curds	75 gm	½ katori
	Assorted vegetables		1½ katori
	Cooking oil	10 gm	2 tsp
Bedtime	Milk	140 ml	1 cup

2200 calorie non-vegetarian meal

Meal	Menu	Weight	Measure
Breakfast	Bread	80 gm	4 slices
	Milk	140 ml	1 cup
	Fruit	100 gm	1 no.
	Butter	6.3 gm	1 tsp
Mid morning snack	Biscuits	20 gm	4 no.
	Fruit	100 gm	1 no.
Lunch	5 Chapaties or		
	Cooked rice	125 gm	
	Daal	25 gm	1 katori

	Curds	75 gm	½ katori
	Assorted vegetables		2 katories
	Cooking oil	15 gm	3 tsp
Tea	Biscuits	20 gm	4 no.
	Fruit	100 gm	1 no.
Dinner	4 Chapaties or		
	Cooked rice	100 gm	
	Meat/Fish		
	Assorted vegetables		1½ katori
	Cooking oil	15 gm	3 tsp
Bedtime	Milk	140 ml	1 cup

Weight reducing diet (1000 calories)

Foods	Include in your diet	Avoid in your diet
Bread	2 slices whole wheat	bread, coffee, cake, waffles
Cereals	none	all
Soups	vegetable, clear broth, bouillon	creamed or thickened soups
Non-veg.	chicken, ham, liver, kidneys	fatty meats, fried meats, fish
Vegetables	up to 12 gm carbohydrates	dried beans, dried peas
Potato	none	all
Fats	2 teaspoons butter or cream	all fats
Fruits	fresh, unsweetened	sweetened, frozen, canned, dried
Sweets	none, except saccharine	all
Beverages	coffee, tea, skim milk	carbonated, whole milk, drinks
Desserts	unsweetened custard, gelatine	cakes, cookies, ice cream, puddings
Miscellaneous	condiments, salts, spices	alcohol, cream sauce, pickles, nuts

Low-salt diet for high BP patients
Do's and don'ts:

○ **Bread:** Include salt-free bread and crackers in your diet. Avoid any bread made with baking soda, salt or baking powder.

○ **Cereals:** Include puffed rice, puffed wheat and broken wheat in your diet. Avoid any other cereal.

○ **Soups:** Include salt-free cream soup in your diet. Avoid soups containing salt.

○ **Non-veg.:** Include freshwater fish (without salt), egg (not more than 1 daily) in your diet. But avoid salted meats, canned meats or fish and glandular meat.

○ **Vegetables:** Any canned, cooked or raw vegetables can be eaten. However, avoid vegetables such as broccoli, Brussels sprouts, cabbage, cauliflower, cucumber, onions, dried peas, green peppers, radish and turnips.

○ **Potato:** Eat potatoes prepared without salt. Avoid fried potatoes and potato chips.

○ **Fats:** Include salt-free butter, cream, lard, oil, salad dressing and vegetable fat. But avoid salted fats.

○ **Fruits:** Include fruit juice, canned/cooked/raw fruit in your diet. But avoid dried fruits.

○ **Desserts:** Include custard, ice cream, unsalted fruit pies and puddings in your diet. Avoid desserts prepared with salt, baking powder, baking soda or egg white.

○ **Sweets:** Include candy, jam, jelly, sugar and syrup in your diet. However, avoid jam or jelly containing sodium benzoate.

○ **Beverages:** Include carbonated beverages, coffee and milk in your diet. Avoid soft water.

○ **Miscellaneous:** Include cocoa (unsalted), cream sauce, herbs, spices, vinegar and unsalted nuts in your diet. Avoid eating chili sauce, ketchup, gravy, mustard, olives, peanut butter, pickles and popcorn.

Low cholesterol (low fat) diet

Foods	Include	Avoid
Bread	any, made without eggs, butter or milk	should not contain milk, eggs
Cereals	any	none
Soups	vegetable, without milk	cream soups, meat soups
Non-veg.	chicken, lean ham, egg white, fish	fatty meats, egg yolk, fry fish
Vegetables	any, cooked without butter or fat	none
Potato	cooked without fat	noodles made with egg
Fats	vegetable cooking oil	animal fat, butter, cream, lard
Fruits	any	none
Sweets	jam, jelly, sugar, hard candy	cream, chocolate, cocoa
Beverages	buttermilk, skim milk, coffee, tea	whole milk, cocoa, chocolate
Miscellaneous	popcorn, salt, spices, vinegar	cream sauce, gravy, popcorn

Low-carbohydrate diet

Foods	Include	Avoid
Bread	2 plain slices	any other type of bread
Cereals	½ cup of cooked cereals in a day	cereals with sugar added
Soups	Bouillon, cream of vegetable	thick soup
Meat	plainly cooked	cooked with excessive gravy
Fats	any, in moderation	none
Fruits	canned or cooked without sugar	canned fruit, dry fruit
Desserts	gelatine sweetened with saccharine	cakes, pastries, ice cream
Sweets	saccharine	all others
Beverages	coffee, tea, milk	carbonated, sweet beverages
Miscellaneous	condiments, spices, vinegar	pickles, cream sauce, ketchup

High calorie diet for underweight

Breads	any, especially whole-grain or enriched bread.
Cereals	any, especially whole-grain or enriched cereal.
Soups	any.
Meat/fish	one egg and two servings of meat.
Vegetables	any, canned, cooked or raw.
Fats	butter, cream, oil, salad dressing.
Fruits	any, canned, cooked, dried or fresh.
Desserts	cakes, cookies, ice cream, pies, puddings.
Sweets	candy, jelly, sugar, others.
Beverages	any, especially those high in calories.
Miscellaneous	condiments, gravy, nuts, salt, spices, vinegar.

Composition of food

Obesity is a major health problem all over the world. Along with poor nutritional habits goes obesity, one of the major problems in our society. Efforts are being made, especially by women, to work out diets to make weight reducing as quick and as easy as possible. Most of the diets rely on reduction of calorie intake and are usually effective only in the short term. Crash diets certainly do this, but they fail to treat nutritional practices as part of the individual's pattern of living. Unless the obese person can alter his or her eating habits, then all efforts will be in vain. Crash dieting without consultation of a doctor or dietician can seriously impair an individual's health irreparably, and sometimes can lead to the extremely serious disorder – anorexia nervosa – a psychiatric illness usually caused by compulsive dieting in women resulting in metabolic disorder. A basic knowledge of some of the common foods and vegetables is given on the following page for easy reference.

Food	Water content	Protein	Fibre	Carbohydrate
Chicken	63%	20%	0	0
Fish	68%	17.5%	0	0
Liver	64%	19%	0	0
Butter	16%	0.5%	0	0.5%
Cheese	4.2%	25%	0	2%
Eggs	74%	12%	0	1%
Bread	36%	7.8%	0	50%
Milk	87%	3.5%	0	4.5%
Rice	12%	7%	1%	77%
Mushrooms	92%	2%	5.5%	0
Potatoes	80%	2%	0.5%	17%
Tomatoes	95%	0.5%	1%	3%
Cabbage	90%	3.5%	1%	5%
Carrot	89%	1.5%	1%	8%
Peas	81%	6%	1.5%	11%
Kidney beans	12%	24%	4.5%	55%
Lettuce	94%	1.5%	1%	3%
Apples	84%	0.5%	2%	13%
Grapefruit	88%	1%	0.5%	10%

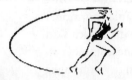

Chapter-12

Programme for Pregnancy and Post-natal Body Care

A little everyday care ensures that the natural beauty of your body does not fade away too soon. Here are a few basic guidelines to a beauty and body regime a woman can maintain during the period of pregnancy and post-natal.

Problems during periods

The changes in the menstrual cycle occur due to female sex hormones from the regulating centre – the pituitary gland, which stimulates ovaries to secrete estrogen hormones. The ovaries begin the secretion of progesterone for the preparation of fertilised egg to settle in the uterus. Due to sudden drop in the level of progesterone and estrogen, the inner lining of uterus (mucus) starts breaking up and escapes out through vagina mixed with blood called as menstrual flow. This changing cycle leaves adverse effect on a woman's appearance. Pigmentation of skin (brownish discolouration of skin) is a major problem during periods and pregnancy. What a woman wants is an even-toned, translucent, radiant and blemish-free skin and slim-trim body during this period. The melanin in the skin is the real culprit. Hyper-pigmentation is usually faced by women during periods, pregnancy and post-natal. The common problems related to pigmentation are usually seen on the face (cheeks, forehead and nose) and other parts on the body, but tend to persist till the delivery of infant and lactating period.

133

Beauty problems during pregnancy

Pregnancy can change your appearance due to rapid hormonal changes, which cause dry, flaky skin or a blotchy acne-prone complexion. Body undergoes many changes including extreme fatness. Skin and body are the first things to bear the brunt. Some of the common problems include very dry, itchy skin, acne and stretch marks all over the body including face. Do not worry, these can be treated during and after pregnancy. Usually, from the second trimester of pregnancy,

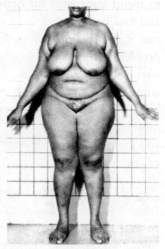

a pregnant woman might suddenly find herself with very dry, taut skin – sand papery to the touch, especially around the stomach, breasts, hands and legs. The fat starts accumulating all over the body. Generally the condition vanishes after delivery. But till then be sure to keep skin extra moisturised with a creamy body lotion. Almond oil or cocoa butter-based creams tend to work wonders in soothing the skin and melting away fat deposits when applied after bath. For some women the skin tends to clear up during pregnancy due to extra blood flow in the system. Acne, pimples and stretch marks are undoubtedly the biggest problems that almost all pregnant women worry about when the skin loses its elasticity due to the stretching of the upper and lower layers of skin. With timely treatment and massage with vitamin E oil accompanied by a balanced diet and simple body movements, the stretch marks may lighten and fatness may be controlled.

The three trimesters of pregnancy

The first three months: There are additional physical strains to cope with along with confusing and conflicting advice from friends and relatives for mother-to-be. In the midst of such pressures, a pregnant woman often has no room for her beauty and body care. But it is very important for an expectant woman to spend some time for herself. If the expectant mother is relaxed and healthy, then her baby stands a good chance of being healthy too. The 40 weeks of pregnancy have several beauty and body problems. An expectant mother may become beautiful, if she starts taking extra care from the very beginning. During the first trimester of pregnancy, there is great hormonal activity in the body. The figure becomes plump and lumpy. The joy to be a mother may be clouded by doubts and disappointment when you look disfigured. Start by thinking positive, as spots appearing on the face, chest or back should not worry you because the increased hormonal activity in your body is causing such temporary upset.

When you are pregnant, pay special attention to lubricate the skin on your stomach, buttocks and breasts. Apply plenty of skin conditioning cream after your bath and rub in baby oil or olive oil every night. Regular lubrication of the skin at this time can pay handsome dividends later on after childbirth. Keep lubricating throughout the nine months of pregnancy. Pay more attention on your diet in this period. You need more nutrients, not more calories. Cut out fried, sweet and fatty foods. If you are non-vegetarian, fish provides the vitamin D you need at this stage. Drink a glass of milk daily, it fulfils the need of calcium. Avoid really strenuous exercise during the crucial first three months. Go to bed early. The most radiant mother-to-be of all is the rested one.

The second trimester: Care taken earlier in the first trimester of pregnancy now begins to pay dividends. Hair and skin conditions improve at this stage. Continue with daily stomach, bottom and breast lubrication. Night cramps are often a problem at this stage. Keep strict watch on your diet and weight gain. Total weight gain during pregnancy should be about 12 kg. Toxaemia (blood poisoning) and high blood pressure are dangers for overweight mothers-to-be, and so are varicose veins. Keep walking (but slowly) with your doctor's advice. It is important to continue light exercise as per your doctor's approval. Going to bed early during this period is a good habit to enhance grooming of your

135

baby in womb. The most comfortable position in bed is lying on your side with one leg slightly in front of the other, one hand under the pillow, and the other by your side to keep weight evenly distributed.

The final months: This is the time for the final preparations to welcome the baby. You will need a lot of energy in the coming months to bring up baby as well as to retain your beauty and posture. Dryness, blotchiness and excessive fat are some of the problems at the end of pregnancy period. Take care to nourish your skin and giving your body plenty of skin cream in the last two months. If you intend to breastfeed your baby, keep your nipples soft with a special cream to help prevent cracking. Massage breasts to avoid over-development and fat. Increase milk and high protein food in your diet. Keep your iron intake high, too. Drink fresh orange juice instead of tea or coffee. A high vitamin C intake helps protect you against infections.

Post-natal care: Having a baby takes a great deal of energy. Even though you have been following a good anti-natal beauty programme, you are bound to feel tired and exhausted for the first few months after the birth of child. Make sure you are having diet rich in nutrients and plenty of vitamin C, protein and minerals. Keep up the iron supplement you took before baby was born. Take care of your body and exercise regularly to become slim.

The pelvis

Before conceiving for the first time, many women are surprisingly unaware of the internal working of their own bodies. However, once the pregnancy is confirmed, the pelvis and its associated muscles and organs become the centre of interest and it is important to understand the role of the pelvis. The bones of the pelvis form the strong frame that acts like a cradle, surrounding, supporting and protecting the womb. The pelvic floor helps to hold the pelvic organs in place. The larger, top ring of pelvic muscle controls the outlets of the urethral and vaginal sphincters. Below the pelvic region is the smaller circle of muscle which contains the stronger anal or rectal sphincter. The overlapping muscles are thicker at the area between the anus and vagina.

Pelvic floor exercises are important throughout your life. If the muscles become slack, there is lack of enjoyment during sexual intercourse as much and a woman may have difficulty reaching orgasm. The male partner will also find love making less enjoyable. A weak pelvic floor can lead to prolapse of uterus and sagging of the walls of vagina.

Pelvis exercises: The following movements will help you prepare the pelvic area for childbirth. Practice the following simple movements in rhythmic slow motion, repeating each for five to six times. This will help provide you the best position for yourself and your baby during labour.

1. **Pelvic tilt (standing position):** The pelvic tilt is an essential movement for maintaining good posture during pregnancy and after the birth. Tilt your pelvis by lifting the pubic bone up in front. The abdominal and buttock muscles are most effectively able to support the trunk and minimise strain on your lower back. To do this exercise, stand resting your back, shoulders and head against the wall. Press your lower back firmly against the wall, pulling in your abdomen and lifting your pubic bone so that your buttocks tighten and leave the wall. Keep shoulders pressed against the wall and move only the pelvis.

2. **Pelvic tilt (second posture):** Kneel with your knees in line with your hips and hands in line with your shoulders. Keeping back flat, pull in your abdominal muscles, tighten your buttocks and do a pelvic tilt, so that your back humps up. Do not rock your pubic bone back in this position.

3. **Dancing exercise:** Dancing is an excellent exercise. Rocking and circling the pelvis are basic movements in all rhythmic dance. You may dance to music either standing or kneeling or on all fours, circling the pelvis. The regular practice of this exercise helps during labour.

137

Spinal exercising

The spine is the supporting structure of the body connecting your head, ribs, pelvis and limbs. Between each movable joint of the spine is a soft jelly-like disc that allows the movement. If you allow your spine to sag, it will cause stiffness and pain. If your back is stiff and inflexible, loosen it up with the exercises as detailed below. Spinal exercises are as following:

- ○ Stretch your spine sitting, standing or lying down. Practice the movement sitting or standing and pressing your back against the wall. Give a pelvic tilt.

- ○ Sit against the wall pressing your back. Now stretch your arms above your head flattening them as far back as you can.

- ○ Kneel with your knees, hip-width apart. Slowly twist to the right, hold for a moment; then repeat to the left. Avoid twisting your hips and thighs.

- ○ Sit cross-legged. Press against your knee to help you twist farther.

- ○ Stand straight, both knees facing forward. Swing your arms for extra momentum and twist from side to side, standing.

How to strengthen your back

'Tailor sitting' strengthens the muscles of back. This position is useful in preparing for labour as it loosens the groin and hips, stretches the muscles of the inner thighs and stimulates the circulation in the lower half of the body. A practice of this posture will help you to hold a variety of positions during labour and will let your legs open wide apart during the delivery of the baby. The following is the procedure for Tailor sitting:

- ○ Sit on the floor with the soles of your feet together. Hold your ankles.

- ○ Bring your pelvis and feet as close together as you can by walking forward on your hips. Keep your back straight.

138

○ In case you feel uncomfortable in practicing this posture, place a couple of cushions under each of your thighs for support.

○ This posture can be performed in lying down position also. Practice Tailor sit posture; then lean backward slowly till your back touches the floor. You can seek the help of your partner while leaning backward and coming to the initial sitting position after a few seconds.

Exercises to strengthen your back

○ Sit against a wall to feel the length of your spine. Lift knees upward so that the soles of both feet press each other. Make sure your back is straight.

○ Sit straight without taking support of wall. Prop yourself up with your arms on the floor to help you lift. Make a loose fist with each hand and press the fist into the floor behind you as you lift your ribs away from the hips. Straighten your back. Make sure, your shoulders do not move up.

How to slim your lower body

In this exercise stretch the groin, inside thighs, back of the legs and the muscles at the front of the thighs. This exercise is particularly important during pregnancy when the extra weight can put undue strain on the knees. The exercise strengthens the muscles and also helps you to cope with the weight of the baby. To practice this exercise, following movements are applied:

○ Sit straight, lifting your back. Spread your legs as much as you can sideways.

○ Tighten the muscles of your legs and keep toes pointing upwards.

○ Now hook big toes with your index and middle fingers. If hands do not touch the feet, take them up to the point you can comfortably.

139

○ Bend forward and rest your forehead or chin on the floor. If it is uncomfortable, do not practice this exercise. Do not bend your knees.

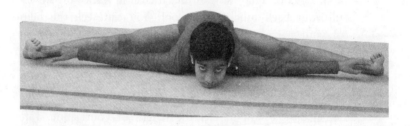

This exercise improves circulation in the pelvic region and makes hamstring muscles elastic. It makes delivery easier and relieves labour pain. The exercise is also especially good for women for curing all menstruation disorders; strengthens genital organs and increases sex power. The exercise keeps joints, muscles, organs and nerves strong and healthy besides slimming the body.

Sagging breasts

Your breasts are likely to become larger and heavier during pregnancy, and unless you support them with a well-fitting bra, they may sag and lose their shape. So even if you don't normally wear a bra, you should do so while your breasts are heavy. There are no muscles in the breasts themselves, but you can help to maintain their shape by exercising the muscle underneath. Here are few exercises/massage movements for breast beauty:

1. Make a loose fist with one hand and clasp the other round it. Hold your hands level with your breasts and press your hands together tightly for few moments. Repeat the sequence several times.

2. Lie on your back. Pull knees up towards the chest without any pull on ankles. Stay in this position for 6-8 seconds, release the knees on the floor and repeat for three to four times. This exercise strengthens the muscles of the

upper part of the body including breasts, relieves lines and wrinkles on waist, abdomen and intestines. Practice of this exercise tones up the muscles of abdomen and intestine, cures constipation and gastric trouble, corrects malfunctioning of stomach, helps uterus come to original position during childbirth. This exercise can also be done in standing position during post-natal, when the knee is pulled up towards the chest without any pull on ankles, one leg at a time. Stay in this position for 6-8 seconds.

3. Massage helps to re-shape your breasts which start expanding during pregnancy and become saggy and shapeless during post-natal when the baby feeds. A regular massage in the bathroom after shower or bath during pregnancy and when the mother is breastfeeding the baby is very helpful to strengthen breast muscle. Start massage making slow, gentle strokes with both hands over the bulge.

Taking care of abdomen during pregnancy

Strong abdominal muscles help you carry the baby more easily without straining your back. They are also helpful during the birth, when the baby is being pushed out; the better the condition of your abdomen muscles, the easier it is to restore them afterward. The following exercises/massage movements help strengthening the abdominal muscles:

○ The most important exercise for the abdomen muscles is simply to pull in your abdomen as you breathe out, as often as you can.

○ **Triangle posture:** is recommended throughout the period of pregnancy, (preferably in the first or second trimester) and after the birth of baby to get rid of flab around the waist and abdomen. Stand with the legs apart. Rotate waist, begin to exhale until the fingers of the right hand touch the ground. Hold for some time, stand up and perform the same movement with the other hand. This posture makes the entire body strong and elastic, and also tones the muscles in the back, hips and legs.

- ○ **Sun exercise:** Stand straight with arms on sides. Raise both arms upward, stretched. Inhale slowly, bend downward and touch the floor with both hands. This posture tones up the muscles of abdomen, waist, hips and relieves extra fat from these areas. The exercise is especially beneficial after the birth of baby.

- ○ **Pawanmukta exercise:** To practice this exercise, lie on your back with your legs bent, feet hip-width apart, hands resting on thighs. Breathe in. As you breathe out raise your head and shoulders, dropping your chin and reaching towards your knees. Sometimes, your shoulders won't lift up smoothly for few days after the birth. Gradually, they will start lifting to hold up for longer periods.

- ○ **Leg roll movement:** This exercise is practiced in the same way as above lying on the back with legs bent, knees together. Lower the knees on the floor and sideways giving movements to the abdomen and legs slowly.

  Posture 2: Side bends: In this movement, lie on your back, legs straight and together with your arms at your sides and palms flat on the thighs. Lift your head and

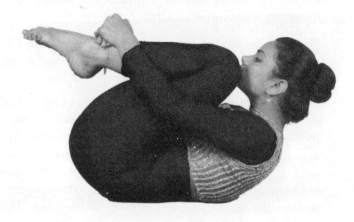

bend to the right. Rest. Lift head and return to the centre. Rest. Lift head and bend to the left and return to the centre after having rest. Repeat the whole process three to four times.

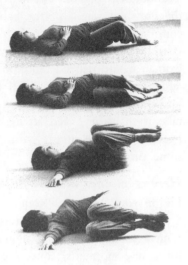

Posture 3: Kneel on movement: Kneel on all fours, your knees in line with your hips and your hands in line with your shoulders. This exercise comprises of stretched leg movements in all directions and walking on all fours. This is a beneficial post-natal exercise.

Abdominal massage is very essential to avoid lines and wrinkles during the third trimester of pregnancy. Start massage from lower abdomen making slow, gentle, circular strokes with both hands over the bulge continuing up to under the breast fold. This is particularly comforting towards the end of pregnancy.

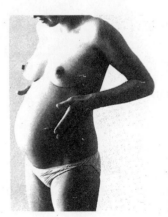
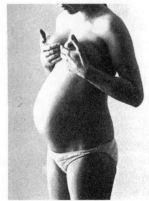

Heavy buttocks

The buttocks play an essential part in supporting the trunk and the growing weight of the baby and abdominal muscles. They control the tilt of your pelvis. As the abdominal muscles become stretched because of the growing bulge in front, a pregnant woman has to depend more on buttocks to keep correct posture and prevent low back pain. If buttocks are flabby and collect a lot of fat, or if they protrude at the sides of your thighs, you can take it that they need strengthening of muscles. The simplest exercise is to squeeze your buttocks together slowly for some time.

Here is another exercise for the buttocks

Lie on your back with your legs bent, feet hip-width apart. Do a pelvic tilt and continue pushing your hips up until your back is in a straight line from shoulders to knees. Hold the position for a few moments, squeezing your buttocks tightly together. Hold for a few seconds, and lower the hips. Repeat three times, twice a day. You can also do this exercise when you are resting on the floor with your legs on a low sofa or bed, keeping the legs straight.

Legs and feet

Unless your legs and feet are strong, the extra weight you are carrying will make you tired resulting cramps and varicose veins. Strong muscles help to prevent cramps, varicose veins and will make your legs feel less sluggish. Exercises that stimulate the blood flow in the nerves are particularly helpful. Here is an exercise to stimulate the nerves of legs:

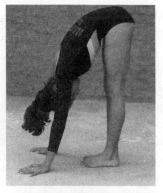

Stand straight with your feet together. Hold on to a wall or a table for balance. Rise up on the balls of your feet. Do a pelvic tilt. Clench your buttocks tightly together. Do several small bends until you are tired. Stand up straight again.

Cramps

These can be very painful and annoying if they wake you up in the middle of the night. There is no proven remedy, but you might try a calcium and vitamin D supplement or extra milk. If you suffer from cramps in the feet, bend it upward. When the cramps subside, do some ankle circles to stimulate the circulation.

Varicose veins

The extra progesterone in your body relaxes the muscles in the walls of your veins, increasing the risk of varicose veins developing. These can appear on the legs or in the vulva (the opening of vagina) or in the anal passage, where they are called haemorrhoids. Take care to avoid constipation in such case. If haemorrhoids is neglected, it can be very painful.

Aching legs

Try to rest with your feet up. Do leg exercises as well. Swimming and walking are both excellent to treat aching legs. Gentle massage up the legs may help and relieve pain.

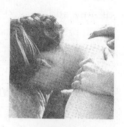

Massaging back

Touching, stroking and holding are the most direct ways of communicating with those you love. During the last stage of pregnancy, you need a massage by your partner with talcum powder, moisturiser or massage oil or on bare skin. Sit on the chair leaning forward on to a cushion. Leaning forward takes the weight of infant in womb, off the lower back. Ask your partner to rest hands on your shoulder and upper back and slide hands downwards on either side of spine. Stroke it slowly and firmly.

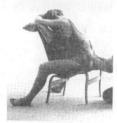

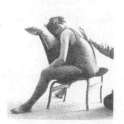

Exercise while taking bath

Have you ever thought of doing exercises in the bathroom which provide pleasant relaxation? A gentle rest in a warm bath with few luxurious simple exercises give very beneficial results. You may have a shower instead of a bath, but you can still do your extra activity there. Warm up between exercises with a warm shower or try doing some of the movements with the water running over you. Make a habit of scrubbing yourself all over as vigorously as possible with a 'loofah' for stimulation of the skin. You also rub off the dead skin always accumulating on the surface. As you sway, twist, and turn, do so as thoroughly and yet as quickly as you can. Quick, deft movements keep your brain in living co-operation with your body. Try to keep washing your own back and feet, even if it is difficult. If you are safe standing on one leg, be sure to do so. This strengthens the muscles of your standing leg and foot, and the muscles of your tummy and back. It keeps the balance centres in your brain. Do not forget to lubricate your joints which strengthen your muscles, keep your brain active and body supple.

Exercise in bed

Exercise can be performed in bed too. These comparatively weightless exercises are beneficial. Never exercise if you are confined to bed with any infection. They are only for those in normal health. Don't attempt to exercise every area each time. For luxurious comfort, have a pillow under each upper arm, which is a most comfortable support for head, neck, back and arms. If possible, lie with no pillows at all. You may find you are more comfortable with a small sausage pillow under your neck. Do not put a pillow into its hollow; instead, put the pillow under your thighs. This relieves the discomfort in your back.

Simple Exercises For New Mothers

Childbirth and care of the newborn are both physically exhausting tasks. Most new mothers find that they do not have the same energy level that they had before their baby was born. In the first few months, the mother's night sleep is disturbed and this adds to the exhaustion. The pressures of taking care of a newborn and managing the house leaves the mother mentally and physically drained. A number of new mothers have found that finding the time to do a few simple exercises increases their energy levels and makes them feel better as well.

Before you join any post-natal exercise class, it is better to consult your doctor and once he has given you a clean chit of health, you can start exercising. Joining an exercise class will not only keep you fit but you will make friends with other new mothers with whom you could form a support group for each other.

Here are a few simple exercises that you could try:

○ **Leg slide:** Lie flat on your back, with your knees bent and feet flat on the floor. Put your hands under your lower back, flat on the ground. While you breathe out, slide your legs gently forward, bringing the knees to the ground. Breathe in and slowly slide your legs up to the starting position.

○ **Pelvic rock:** Lie on your back with your knees bent and feet flat on the floor. While breathing out move your pelvis in a rocking movement so that your lower back is flat on the floor. Then move your pelvis again so that your lower back is lifted from the floor.

○ **Pelvic floor exercises:** Contract your vagina in the same way as you would to stop yourself from passing urine and count till four. Then relax; you should feel the difference between the two positions. Repeat this exercise in set of six several times a day. Contract and relax your vagina in quick succession. Breathe normally while doing these exercises.

Start exercising at the earliest after delivery, even if you have had a Caesarean section. Exercising will improve circulation and aid in healing. Begin slowly in the initial weeks after childbirth. Do not lie flat on your back and lift both your legs in the air. Do not do sit-ups.

Exercises sitting on a chair
Abdominal and back exercises

The movements given below help to shorten and tighten up the abdominal muscles in all directions:

○ **Waist side bends:** This exercise movement stretches and strengthens the muscles at the side of the trunk, back and front. It mobilises the five joints of the lower back. Clasp the hands just above the head, elbows out sideways. Do a three-point pull. Bend sideways to the right as far as you can, keeping the pelvis firmly on the chair. Hold the position for a few seconds. Return to initial standing 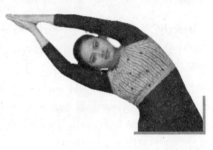 position and repeat on other side. Do not allow the chest to sag or rotate. This exercise tones up abdominal and back muscles, and slims the waist.

○ **Waist twist:** Tones up and mobilises the diagonal muscles and joints of the abdomen, upper back and the neck. Place the hands flat on the upper chest. Twist round to the left, turning your head as far as you can. The pelvis must remain facing forwards. Go on pressing round in small further movements, with the head and upper body. Face front again and repeat to the other side. Try not to lift the shoulders.

○ **Waist diagonal bend:** It mobilises the whole spine. Tones up abdominal and back muscles. Sit on a chair or a stool. Clasp hands just above the head, elbows out sideways. Twist to the left as far as you can. Return to starting position and repeat on right side. Do this exercise

148

three to four times. Do not attempt this exercise if you have any weakness or pain in the lower back.

○ **The pelvic tilt:** Sit on a chair near the front of the seat, hands holding the back. Start rolling the pelvis so that the pubic bone comes up. Straighten the curve of the lower back so that the tummy is compressed. Return to the starting position after 10-15 counts. This exercise helps easy movement of pelvis and mobilises hip joints and lower back. Keep upright from the waist while doing exercise.

Buttock exercise

This exercise is particularly applicable to women who usually have more fat around the buttocks after delivery of child. Sit correctly on chair or a stool. Move the feet slightly forwards, hands resting on the upper chest. Then do a pelvic tilt pressing the thighs downwards and rotating them outwards. Repeat several times and stop when you feel uncomfortable.

Thighs and hips exercises

Tighten the front of thighs, that increases the circulation in the muscles of thighs and hips. Sit on a chair or a stool with hand on hips. Do a pelvic tilt and turn the thighs outwards. Left foot should remain on the ground during exercise, whereas lift right leg off the floor, knees slightly bent and foot bent upwards. Now straighten the right leg quickly and start kicks, pushing the heel away from you. Repeat the kick several times until the leg begins to tire. Return to the starting position and repeat exercise with the other leg. If you have painful knees, leave out this exercise or gently bend and stretch the leg instead of kicking.

Exercises lying on the floor

Exercises to strengthen the muscles of back

Sit on the floor with legs bent, knees dropped outwards and the soles of the feet together. Clasp hands around the toes and press soles of both feet. If you are feeling uncomfortable, put a cushion under your bottom and hold the ankles instead of the toes.

Press the knees towards the floor. Straighten the back, lifting the chest. This exercise leaves the following effects:

(i) Strengthens the back muscles.

(ii) Mobilises the hip joints.

(iii) Stretches the Inward Rotators and Abductors of the hips.

Exercises to stretch thigh muscles

Sit on the floor with the legs as far apart and straight as reasonably comfortable. Knees caps should face upwards. Loosely fist the hands and press them on the floor behind. This posture strengthens the back muscles, mobilises the hip joints and stretches inside thigh muscles.

To stretch the muscles on the back of the thighs and back of lower legs, sit on the floor with legs spread straight forwards, feet together pointing upwards towards the face. Loosely fist the hands and press them on the floor behind. Put a cushion under your bottom and bend your knees a little if you find this position difficult. This exercise also helps to strengthen back muscles and mobilise the hip joints.

Back control muscle exercise

Sit on the floor with legs spread straight forwards. Place a towel around the middle of the feet and hold it in both hands. Pull the towel and lower the trunk slowly forwards, keeping the back straight and the chest lifted. Hold the position for at least 30 seconds. Repeat this exercise for a few times. Inhale as you lift trunk, exhale as you lower the trunk. Finally lower the trunk and clasp the hands under the feet to relax. Women should do this exercise without any pressure.

Pelvic exercise

Lie on the floor straight. Bend the knees up, keeping feet flat on the floor, hip-width apart. Roll the pelvis so that the pubic bone in front comes up towards your nose. Your lower back will press onto the floor and your tummy will be compressed. Let the pelvis roll back to the starting position. Repeat as often as you can do without discomfort. Breathe in when starting the position, breathe out as you tilt the pelvis upwards and breathe normally as you hold the position. Breathe in as the pelvis rolls back to starting position. Keep the shoulders down away from the ears and the top half of the body quite at ease.

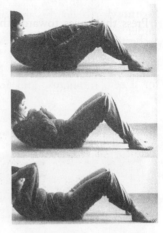

For mobilising the joints of the lumbar region (lower back), tighten muscles at the sides of the waist. Do not lift the hips off the floor as you work. Only move the legs as a result of the action by the pelvis. This exercise is particularly helpful for those who tend to get stiff in the lower back, especially after sleep. This exercise can also be done while standing, and lifting the pelvis. The exercise is very useful if you have to stand for long periods.

Leg-raising exercise for thighs and buttocks

Posture-1: Lie on your right side with the body and legs in a straight line. Keeping both knees facing forwards, lift left leg up until the pelvis begins to lift sideways. Hold the position for ten seconds. Lower the leg slowly and let the leg rest on the floor. Hold for ten seconds and repeat as often as you can do comfortably. Now roll over and repeat the sequence on the other side.

Posture-2: Lie on your right side as in case of Posture 1. Lift the left leg up to about ten inches off the floor at an angle of 45 degrees. Swing lifted leg back and turn it out allowing the chest and pelvis to come forward a little. Lower the leg to the floor. Now repeat the sequence on the other side. This exercise can also be done standing. Do not arch or hollow the back.

Leg-raising exercise for toning the loose muscles of buttocks and thighs

Women, soon after childbirth, should avoid this exercise for at least two to three weeks.

Posture-1: To do this exercise, lie on the tummy with a cushion under the pelvis. Bend the elbows and put the hands in front of you on the floor. Rest your forehead on the hands. Now raise both legs, trying to lift the thighs off the floor. Hold the position for a few moments, and lower the legs gently to the floor.

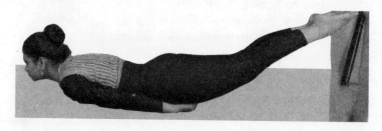

Position-2: Perform this exercise as in case of Posture-1 except taking the legs apart. Make small circles clockwise, then anti-clockwise with the legs at the hip joints. Breathing should be normal. Do not hold the breath. If your legs are weak, lift only one leg at a time. If this exercise hurts your back, do not perform it.

Stretching the muscles of the back and neck

Kneel on the ground. Rest your bottom on or near the heel. Curl forwards and tuck your head in towards your knees. Pull your shoulders down and rest the hands, palms up, on the floor on sides. Rest in this position for as long as you like.

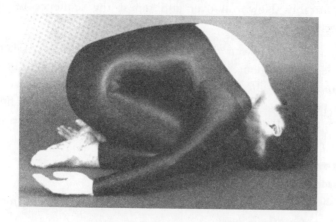

DETOX – to eliminate toxins and get rid of extra fat after childbirth

Daily care can help keep your whole body smooth and soft. But during periods, pregnancy and after delivering child, many times specific problems, usually accumulation of flesh on various parts on the body, arise which need particular attention. Detoxification is the best way to eliminate toxins, get radiant skin and get rid of extra fat. Better seek the advice of your doctor before starting practice.

- If you are overweight.
- Fat has accumulated on visible parts of your body and breasts.
- You have cellulite.
- The skin looks bumpy on upper arms.
- Your body feels no energy and you have poor circulation.
- Your skin on the face and body is very dry and looks chalky.
- Your skin looks grey and lifeless.
- You have dark circles and puffiness around the eyes.
- You are getting breakouts on the face and body.

The following are easy ways to detox to beautify and slim down:

Massage

It leaves a miraculous effect to improve circulation and lymph drainage to banish cellulite.

Aroma treatment

Massaging fatty parts of the body with Aroma oils, mixing up about five drops of pure essential oil (such as lemon, juniper) with 10 ml of a carrier oil (preferably sweet almond oil) is very useful to melt fat. Massage as long as it takes the oil to be absorbed on the areas of body such as your hips, butt, thighs and abdomen once a day.

153

Spa massage

It helps to improve circulation if applied after a bath while the skin is still damp and warm. Mix to the massage oil a body contouring cream (readily available in the market) for better and smoothing results.

Body brush

It is excellent treatment for busting cellulite, which smoothes and firms the skin. Do not neglect your back. Brush your back, legs and arms towards your heart in a circular, clockwise movement through your tummy (which is worst affected with extra flesh and wrinkles after childbirth).

Face and body masking

Masking is a good flush out and helps to clear a congested skin using stimulating herbal ingredients such as rosemary and eucalyptus, which leave dehydrating effect on dry as well as oily skins. Mask your skin for 5 to 20 minutes depending upon the condition, use wet packs which help to lower high temperature, raise a subnormal temperature, relieve inner congestion, promote elimination, stimulate sluggish circulation – all these help to shed off extra fat.

Steam bath

Also known as Sauna Bath, it is one of the most important water treatments which induces perspiration. Sauna helps losing a couple of kilos, but you will put them again if you eat or drink immediately after having bath. Do not drink anything for at least one hour after the bath. Steam bath (sauna) along with exercise and good diet can do wonders in reducing weight. To exercise 15 minutes in sauna is equivalent to running two kilometres. Toxins are eliminated through the skin in sauna bath, which helps clearing cellulite besides curing many skin problems like acne, dull and lifeless complexion. Always seek advice of a doctor before starting sauna bath as it may leave harmful effects if started immediately after the delivery of baby.

Hip baths

Hip bath is one of the most useful forms of hydrotherapy, where a bath is taken in a tub filled with water which involves only the hips and the abdominal region. The water level in the tub covers the hips up to the navel when the patient sits in it. Hip bath is taken in cold, hot, neutral water having alternate temperature. Rub the abdomen briskly from navel downwards and across the body with a coarse wet cloth for excellent results in eliminating obesity. Such baths help to reduce extra flesh from the hips and abdomen. Consult a naturopath before having hip bath after childbirth.

Cold Hip Bath is taken for 30 minutes in water having temperature varying between 10-15 degrees C. *Hot Hip Bath* is taken for eight to ten minutes at water temperature 40-45 degrees C. Do not apply friction to the abdomen in this bath. *Cold & Hot Hip Bath* is a treatment in which the patient sits in the hot tub (water temperature 40-45 degrees C.) for five minutes, followed by a cold bath (water temperature 10-18 degrees C.) for three minutes. This bath relieves chronic inflammatory conditions of the pelvic region, and cellulite. These hip baths are very useful in fighting obesity, and relieve constipation, indigestion, diarrhoea, dysentery, and cure uterine problems such as irregular menstruation, uterine infection, pelvic inflammation, piles, hepatic congestion, ovarian displacement, dilation of stomach and colon, haemorrhage of the bladder and many other problems which affect beauty and body.

Lymphatic drainage therapy

This therapy needs gentle pressure on the lymphatic system to move waste materials out of the body quickly. These waste materials are drained out through urine and relieve cellulite.

Sandalwood treatment

It is best suited for water retention, is diuretic and diaphoretic and leads to detoxification. It triggers skin to sweat and release toxins, and act as a disinfectant. Sandalwood unlocks trapped fluid and toxins stored in the tissues, which helps reduce fatness in the body.

155

Panchkarma Massage

Panchkarma means '5 actions', which is an ancient scientific system for detoxification and rejuvenates the whole body system. It relieves stress on the muscles and internal organs, balances body, mind and soul. Vigorous and gentle rhythmic soothing movements applied on the body help to achieve maximum results in burning fat.

Shiatsu therapy

This therapy is also known as acupressure. There are nearly 600 Shiatsu Points on the human body. Pressure on these points with both hands moving rhythmically along the meridians from one point to the other, pressing each from three to seven seconds, produce energy that flows in the body and improve the circulation and induce relaxation. Shiatsu therapy is a wide subject, but here only a couple of tips are being given, which help to reduce fat.

1. When pressing on front abdominal area, at one inch either side of the navel, reduces fat accumulated in the belly area besides stimulating and energising the muscles of abdomen.

2. When pressing on the front abdominal area, at three inches below the navel, helps weight reduction and cures cellulite.

Surya mudra

This 'mudra' helps in reducing body fat. Bend the ring finger and press it with the tip of thumb for 10 to 15 minutes daily in the morning and in the evening. Perform this mudra preferably sitting in Yoga posture — *Padma Asana*. Start practicing after a month of delivery of child.

These exercises performed regularly will surely help in getting rid of excess fat and gaining a slim-trim body after childbirth.

Safe-n-Sure Weight Loss Programme

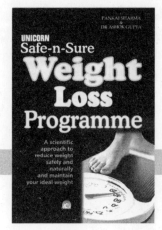

Pankaj Sharma &
Dr. Ashok Gupta

This self-help weight loss book is probably India's *first well-defined programme on losing weight positively and naturally.* The book includes information on other weight loss regimens in the market and discusses their pitfalls.

Following the *Safe-n-Sure Weight Loss Programme* also ensures you don't regain the lost weight after some time. This step-by-step programme includes an exercise regimen and crucial information on food and diet, with an exclusive chapter on low-calorie recipes, vegetarian as well as non-vegetarian. All of which makes this book a truly holistic weight loss guide that will help you lose weight *safely* and *naturally,* and *maintain* your ideal weight thereafter.

Demy Size • Pages: 132
Price: Rs. 96/- • Postage: Rs. 15/-

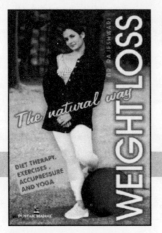

Weight Loss
—The Natural Way

Shed Your Weight
without Tears

Dr. Rajeshwari

*T*oday everyone is health and fitness conscious, regardless of age and sex. As a result, a number of health clubs and slimming centres have mushroomed to cater to the health conscious people.

But obesity does not always respond to crash diets and rigourous exercises, which in addition to being expensive may not suit everyone.

This is because there are several causes of obesity and it differs from person to person. The main causes are faulty food habits, consumption of junk food and lack of exercise or activity. Natural treatment, with proper diet as its base, combined with exercise is the only method of getting rid of unwanted fat and keeping it off.

Weight Loss—The Natural Way is aimed at those who would like to treat themselves naturally through the simple methods given. The aim of the book is to wean people away from harmful eating patterns and foods by giving them natural and healthy substitutes.

The book helps people to control obesity through:
❖ Yoga ❖ Acupuncture ❖ Acupressure ❖ Water Cure

Demy Size • Pages: 96
Price: Rs. 80/- • Postage: Rs. 15/-

Slim & Smart Body

A Fitness Programme for Men & Women

Barun Roy

*O*besity is a worldwide phenomenon with the increasing use of modern gadgets and conveniences, which ensure we do not have to move a muscle except to press the remote button! The burgeoning incidences of disease, depression and premature deaths have meant a rising awareness about the benefits of exercise.

With most exercise regimens making adherents huff and puff, people usually fall by the wayside before the benefits are noticeable. But relax! This book does not expect you to cross the pain barrier. Instead, the focus is on a practical, pleasant and doable exercise regimen where you tailor each programme to suit your individual requirements.

In essence, this book will ensure that exercise is no longer a word you dread, but something you look forward to. The myriad benefits will thereafter flow of their own accord. And a fit, active, healthy life will be your ultimate reward.

Demy Size • Pages: 156
Price: Rs. 80/- • Postage: Rs. 15/-